Psychosocial Interventions for Mental and Substance Use Disorders

A Framework for Establishing Evidence-Based Standards

Committee on Developing Evidence-Based Standards for
Psychosocial Interventions for Mental Disorders

Board on Health Sciences Policy

Mary Jane England, Adrienne Stith Butler, Monica L. Gonzalez, *Editors*

INSTITUTE OF MEDICINE
OF THE NATIONAL ACADEMIES

THE NATIONAL ACADEMIES PRESS
Washington, D.C.
www.nap.edu

THE NATIONAL ACADEMIES PRESS   500 Fifth Street, NW   Washington, DC 20001

NOTICE: The project that is the subject of this report was approved by the Governing Board of the National Research Council, whose members are drawn from the councils of the National Academy of Sciences, the National Academy of Engineering, and the Institute of Medicine. The members of the committee responsible for the report were chosen for their special competences and with regard for appropriate balance.

This study was supported by Contract No. 10001728 between the National Academy of Sciences and the National Institutes of Health, Contract No. 10001759 between the National Academy of Sciences and the U.S. Department of Veterans Affairs, and Contract No. 10001803 between the National Academy of Sciences and the U.S. Department of Health and Human Services, and grants from the American Psychiatric Association, American Psychological Association, Association for Behavioral Health and Wellness, and the National Association of Social Workers. Any opinions, findings, conclusions, or recommendations expressed in this publication are those of the author(s) and do not necessarily reflect the views of the organizations or agencies that provided support for the project.

International Standard Book Number-13: 978-0-309-31694-1
International Standard Book Number-10: 0-309-31694-4
Library of Congress Control Number: 2015948348

Additional copies of this report are available for sale from the National Academies Press, 500 Fifth Street, NW, Keck 360, Washington, DC 20001; (800) 624-6242 or (202) 334-3313; http://www.nap.edu.

For more information about the Institute of Medicine, visit the IOM home page at: www.iom.edu.

Printed in the United States of America

The serpent has been a symbol of long life, healing, and knowledge among almost all cultures and religions since the beginning of recorded history. The serpent adopted as a logotype by the Institute of Medicine is a relief carving from ancient Greece, now held by the Staatliche Museen in Berlin.

Suggested citation: IOM (Institute of Medicine). 2015. *Psychosocial interventions for mental and substance use disorders: A framework for establishing evidence-based standards*. Washington, DC: The National Academies Press.

"Knowing is not enough; we must apply.
Willing is not enough; we must do."
—Goethe

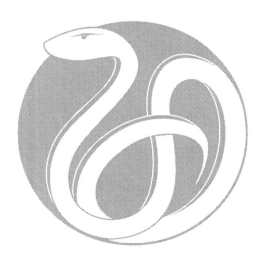

INSTITUTE OF MEDICINE
OF THE NATIONAL ACADEMIES

Advising the Nation. Improving Health.

THE NATIONAL ACADEMIES
Advisers to the Nation on Science, Engineering, and Medicine

The **National Academy of Sciences** is a private, nonprofit, self-perpetuating society of distinguished scholars engaged in scientific and engineering research, dedicated to the furtherance of science and technology and to their use for the general welfare. Upon the authority of the charter granted to it by the Congress in 1863, the Academy has a mandate that requires it to advise the federal government on scientific and technical matters. Dr. Ralph J. Cicerone is president of the National Academy of Sciences.

The **National Academy of Engineering** was established in 1964, under the charter of the National Academy of Sciences, as a parallel organization of outstanding engineers. It is autonomous in its administration and in the selection of its members, sharing with the National Academy of Sciences the responsibility for advising the federal government. The National Academy of Engineering also sponsors engineering programs aimed at meeting national needs, encourages education and research, and recognizes the superior achievements of engineers. Dr. C. D. Mote, Jr., is president of the National Academy of Engineering.

The **Institute of Medicine** was established in 1970 by the National Academy of Sciences to secure the services of eminent members of appropriate professions in the examination of policy matters pertaining to the health of the public. The Institute acts under the responsibility given to the National Academy of Sciences by its congressional charter to be an adviser to the federal government and, upon its own initiative, to identify issues of medical care, research, and education. Dr. Victor J. Dzau is president of the Institute of Medicine.

The **National Research Council** was organized by the National Academy of Sciences in 1916 to associate the broad community of science and technology with the Academy's purposes of furthering knowledge and advising the federal government. Functioning in accordance with general policies determined by the Academy, the Council has become the principal operating agency of both the National Academy of Sciences and the National Academy of Engineering in providing services to the government, the public, and the scientific and engineering communities. The Council is administered jointly by both Academies and the Institute of Medicine. Dr. Ralph J. Cicerone and Dr. C. D. Mote, Jr., are chair and vice chair, respectively, of the National Research Council.

www.national-academies.org

SARAH HUDSON SCHOLLE, Vice President of Research and Analysis, National Committee for Quality Assurance

JOHN T. WALKUP, Professor of Psychiatry, DeWitt Wallace Senior Scholar, Vice Chair of Psychiatry, and Director, Division of Child and Adolescent Psychiatry, Department of Psychiatry, Weill Cornell Medical College, Cornell University

MYRNA WEISSMAN, Diane Goldman Kempner Family Professor of Epidemiology and Psychiatry, Columbia University College of Physicians and Surgeons; Chief, Division of Epidemiology, New York State Psychiatric Institute

IOM Staff

ADRIENNE STITH BUTLER, Study Director
MONICA L. GONZALEZ, Associate Program Officer
THELMA L. COX, Administrative Assistant
LORA K. TAYLOR, Financial Associate
ANDREW M. POPE, Director, Board on Health Sciences Policy

Consultants

GARY BOND, Professor of Psychiatry, Dartmouth University
RONA BRIERE, Editor
BRUCE CHORPITA, Professor of Psychology, University of California, Los Angeles
MIRIAM DAVIS, Writer

Reviewers

This report has been reviewed in draft form by individuals chosen for their diverse perspectives and technical expertise, in accordance with procedures approved by the National Research Council's Report Review Committee. The purpose of this independent review is to provide candid and critical comments that will assist the institution in making its published report as sound as possible and to ensure that the report meets institutional standards for objectivity, evidence, and responsiveness to the study charge. The review comments and draft manuscript remain confidential to protect the integrity of the deliberative process. We wish to thank the following individuals for their review of this report:

Margarita Alegría, Harvard Medical School
Floyd E. Bloom, The Scripps Research Institute
Robert Drake, Dartmouth Psychiatric Research Center
Deborah Finfgeld-Connett, University of Missouri
Russell E. Glasgow, University of Colorado School of Medicine
Carol D. Goodheart, Independent Practice
George Isham, HealthPartners Institute for Education and Research
Ned H. Kalin, University of Wisconsin
Eric M. Plakun, The Austen Riggs Center
Scott L. Rauch, McLean Hospital
Richard Saitz, Boston University School of Public Health
Rusty Selix, California Council of Community Mental Health
    Agencies

Shelley E. Taylor, University of California, Los Angeles
John R. Weisz, Harvard University

Although the reviewers listed above provided many constructive comments and suggestions, they were not asked to endorse the report's conclusions or recommendations, nor did they see the final draft of the report before its release. The review of this report was overseen by **Huda Akil,** University of Michigan, and **Alan F. Schatzberg,** Stanford University School of Medicine. Appointed by the National Research Council and the Institute of Medicine, they were responsible for making certain that an independent examination of this report was carried out in accordance with institutional procedures and that all review comments were carefully considered. Responsibility for the final content of this report rests entirely with the authoring committee and the institution.

Preface

Although a wide range of evidence-based psychosocial interventions are currently in use, most consumers of mental health care find it difficult to know whether they are receiving high-quality care. Providers represent many different disciplines and types of facilities, the delivery of care is fragmented, interventions are supported by varying levels of scientific evidence, performance metrics may or may not be used to measure the quality of care delivered, and insurance coverage determinations are not standardized. In this report, the Institute of Medicine's Committee on Developing Evidence-Based Standards for Psychosocial Interventions for Mental Disorders offers a framework for use by the behavioral health field in developing efficacy standards for psychosocial interventions.

Together with the Mental Health Parity and Addiction Equity Act of 2008, the Patient Protection and Affordable Care Act of 2010 (ACA) will significantly expand access to high-quality interventions for mental health/substance use disorders. In this opportune context, the committee began its work by defining psychosocial interventions for such disorders in a way that is applicable across populations, providers, and settings. The committee recommends that psychosocial interventions be elevated to a position of equal regard with physical health care, that the measurement and improvement strategies used in mental health care likewise be equated with those used in physical health care, and that the importance of context and infrastructure for high-quality psychosocial interventions receive greater emphasis.

The committee envisions a bold path forward for the behavioral health field within the framework presented in this report for applying and strengthening the evidence base for psychosocial interventions. In this framework, the committee recommends that psychosocial interventions be considered in terms of their elements of therapeutic change, and that these elements be subject to systematic reviews, quality measurement, and quality improvement efforts. Key to the framework are a consumer-centered approach to care and the continuous need to strengthen the evidence base. Above all, the committee strove to propose a path forward in which the roles of scientific evidence and quality improvement would be afforded the same importance in mental health care that they have in physical health care.

The committee is most grateful to the sponsors of this study for entrusting us with the opportunity to develop this timely report. As committee chair, I am also deeply appreciative of the expert work of our dedicated, hard-working, and collegial committee members and their forward-thinking approach. Study director Adrienne Stith Butler offered superb leadership, with instrumental support from Monica Gonzalez and Thelma Cox. Andrew Pope also offered exceptional guidance. It is the committee's hope that this report will assist not only payers, purchasers, and providers in their vital efforts to bring high-quality, evidence-based psychosocial interventions into clinical practice, but also the broader consumer community, whose members should be involved in and benefit from each step of the framework offered in this report.

Mary Jane England, *Chair*
Committee on Developing Evidence-Based Standards
for Psychosocial Interventions for Mental Disorders

Acknowledgments

The committee and staff are indebted to a number of individuals and organizations that made important contributions to the study process and this report. The committee wishes to thank these individuals, but recognizes that attempts to identify all and acknowledge their contributions would require more space than is available in this brief section.

To begin, the committee would like to thank the sponsors of this report. Funding for this study was provided by the American Psychiatric Association, American Psychological Association, Association for Behavioral Health and Wellness, National Association of Social Workers, National Institutes of Health, the Office of the Assistant Secretary for Planning and Evaluation within the U.S. Department of Health and Human Services, Substance Abuse and Mental Health Services Administration, and the U.S. Department of Veterans Affairs.

The committee gratefully acknowledges the contributions of the many individuals who provided valuable input to its work. These individuals helped the committee understand varying perspectives on quality measurement and improvement of psychosocial interventions. In particular, the committee is grateful for the time and effort of those who provided important information and data at its open workshops; Appendix A lists these individuals and their affiliations. The committee is also grateful for the contributions of Alisa Decatur and Heather Lee.

Finally, many within the Institute of Medicine were helpful to the study staff. The committee would like to thank Laura DeStefano, Chelsea Aston Frakes, and Greta Gorman for their invaluable assistance.

Contents

APPENDIXES

Boxes, Figures, and Tables

BOXES

FIGURES

TABLES

Acronyms

ABPN	American Board of Psychiatry and Neurology
ACA	Patient Protection and Affordable Care Act
ACGME	Accreditation Council for Graduate Medical Education
ACO	accountable care organization
ACS	Adult Consumer Satisfaction Survey
ACT	assertive community treatment
AHRQ	Agency for Healthcare Research and Quality
ASPE	Assistant Secretary for Planning and Evaluation
CAHPS	Consumer Assessment of Healthcare Providers and Systems
CBT	cognitive-behavioral therapy
CF	cystic fibrosis
CHIP	Children's Health Insurance Program
CHIPRA	Children's Health Insurance Program Reauthorization Act
CMS	Centers for Medicare & Medicaid Services
CPT	Current Procedural Terminology
DALY	disability-adjusted life-year
DMM	Distillation and Matching Model
DoD	U.S. Department of Defense
EBP	evidence-based practice
EHR	electronic health record
EMDR	eye movement desensitization and reprocessing

EPC	Evidence-Based Practice Center
EPOC	Cochrane Effective Practice and Organization of Care Group
ESP	Evidence-Based Synthesis Program
FDA	U.S. Food and Drug Administration
FFS	fee-for-service
GRADE	Grading of Recommendations, Assessment, Development and Evaluation
HHS	U.S. Department of Health and Human Services
HIPAA	Health Insurance Portability and Accountability Act
HITECH	Health Information Technology for Economic and Clinical Health Act
HMO	health maintenance organization
HRSA	Health Resources and Services Administration
IAPT	Improving Access to Psychological Therapies
ICD	International Classification of Diseases
IOM	Institute of Medicine
IPT	interpersonal therapy
MAP	Measures Application Partnership
MH/SU	mental health and substance use
MHPAEA	Mental Health Parity and Addiction Equity Act
MHRN	Mental Health Research Network
MHSIP	Mental Health Statistics Improvement Program
ML	machine learning
NAS	National Academy of Sciences
NASW	National Association of Social Workers
NCQA	National Committee for Quality Assurance
NHS	National Health Service of the United Kingdom
NIAAA	National Institute on Alcohol Abuse and Alcoholism
NICE	National Institute for Health and Care Excellence of the United Kingdom
NIDA	National Institute on Drug Abuse
NIMH	National Institute of Mental Health
NQF	National Quality Forum
NREPP	National Registry of Evidence-based Programs and Practices
NSP	National Standard Project

P4P	pay-for-performance
PAR	participatory action research
PCORI	Patient-Centered Outcomes Research Institute
PCORnet	National Patient-Centered Clinical Research Network
PCPI	Physician Consortium for Performance Improvement
PICOT	population/disease, intervention or variable of interest, comparison, outcome, time
RAS	Recovery Assessment Scale
RCT	randomized controlled trial
SAMHSA	Substance Abuse and Mental Health Services Administration
SMRS	Scientific Merit Rating Scale
VA	U.S. Department of Veterans Affairs
VHA	Veterans Health Administration
WHO	World Health Organization
YFS	Youth and Family Satisfaction Survey

Glossary[1]

ACA: The Patient Protection and Affordable Care Act (ACA), known colloquially as health care reform or "Obamacare," was designed to increase the quality and affordability of health care for all Americans. The law's provisions focus on expanding coverage, controlling health care costs, and improving the health care delivery system (KFF, 2013). The law became effective on March 23, 2010. Several major provisions, including the individual mandate, guaranteed access to insurance for those with preexisting conditions, minimum standards for health insurance policies, federal subsidies, and the implementation of health insurance exchanges, were phased in through 2014.[2]

Accreditation: "A voluntary process by which a nongovernmental agency grants a time-limited recognition to an institution, organization, or business, or other entity after verifying that it has met predetermined and standardized criteria" (McHugh et al., 2014, p. 2; NOCA, 2005, p. 5).

Certification: "The voluntary process by which a nongovernmental entity grants a time-limited recognition and use of a credential to an individual after verifying that he or she has met predetermined and standardized criteria. It is the vehicle that a profession or occupation uses to differentiate among its members, using standards, sometimes developed through a consensus-

---

[1] Definitions for terms without a citation were developed by the committee.
[2] Patient Protection and Affordable Care Act (ACA), Public Law 111-148, 111th Congress, 1st session (March 23, 2010).

driven process, based on existing legal and psychometric requirements" (McHugh et al., 2014, p. 2; NOCA, 2005, p. 5).

Clinical practice guidelines: "Statements that include recommendations intended to optimize patient care that are informed by a systematic review of evidence and assessment of the benefits and harms of clinical interventions in particular circumstances" (IOM, 2011, p. 25).

Clinical trial: "A clinical trial is a prospective biomedical or behavioral research study of human subjects that is designed to answer specific questions about biomedical or behavioral interventions (vaccines, drugs, treatments, devices, or new ways of using known drugs, treatments, or devices). Clinical trials are used to determine whether new biomedical or behavioral interventions are safe, efficacious, and effective" (The Bill & Melinda Gates Foundation, 2015).

Comparative effectiveness research: "The generation and synthesis of evidence to compare the benefits and harms of alternative methods for preventing, diagnosing, treating, and monitoring a clinical condition or improving the delivery of care" (IOM, 2009, p. 41).

Competency: A skill or capability that is developed or measured by credentialing programs. Examples of competencies include psychomotor skills and complex cognitive skills; practice-based learning and improvement; communication and clinical skills; patient care and care coordination; professionalism; system-based practice; medical knowledge; and knowledge, skills, and attitudes (Holmboe, 2014; Lauzon Clabo, 2014; Needleman et al., 2014).

Consumers: People with mental illnesses and/or chemical dependency who receive services in settings where it is not customary to use the term "patient." These settings would include, for example, outpatient and community-based mental health, residential, and psychosocial settings. The term "consumer" has been applied to people with disabilities who are organizing to be treated as consumers in health care rather than plan enrollees in an insurance company. A consumer is thus someone who strives to be treated like a buyer, with rights to information regarding insurance and treatment. Consumers have organized into peer-run networks and through research and evaluation efforts supported by the Substance Abuse and Mental Health Services Administration (SAMHSA).

Credentialing: "Processes used to designate that an individual, programme, institution or product has met established standards set by an agent (governmental or nongovernmental) recognised as qualified to carry out this task. The standards may be minimal and mandatory or above the minimum and voluntary" (International Council of Nurses, 2009, p. 1; Needleman et al., 2014, p. 1). These standards should be defined, published, psychometrically sound, legally defensible, and uniformly tested. The qualified agent should provide objective, third-party assessments (Hickey et al., 2014; McHugh et al., 2014; NOCA, 2005; U.S. Department of Labor, 2014). The purpose of credentialing is to protect the public, enable and enforce professional accountability, and support quality practice and services (Newhouse, 2014).

Delphi method/technique: A series of sequential questionnaires or "rounds," interspersed with controlled feedback, aimed at gaining the most reliable consensus of opinion of an "expert panel" (Powell, 2003). The technique is intended to correct for a lack of conclusive data by drawing on and sharing the knowledge and experience of experts (Fink et al., 1984).

Effect size: The difference between treatment and control groups, generally expressed in standard deviation units.

Effectiveness: The benefit of an intervention under real-world conditions.

Efficacy: The benefit of an intervention under the ideal circumstances of a randomized controlled clinical trial.

Element: A therapeutic activity, technique, or strategy, categorized as either nonspecific or specific. Nonspecific elements are fundamental strategies of engagement that occur in most if not all psychosocial interventions (e.g., a trusting relationship with a therapist). Specific elements are unique to a particular theoretical orientation and approach (e.g., systematic exposure to feared objects is a specific element of cognitive-behavioral therapy for anxiety).

External validity: "The extent to which the results of a study can be generalized to other situations and to other populations" (Brewer, 2000, p. 4).

Family: "Not only people related by blood or marriage, but also close friends, partners, companions, and others whom patients would want as part of their care team" (IOM, 2015, p. 28).

Fee-for-service: "A payment system in which a health care program or plan pays providers a fee for each covered service performed for its enrollees" (CBO, 2013, p. 41).

Fidelity: The degree to which a given psychosocial intervention is implemented as intended in research studies.

Functional ability: An individual's actual or potential capacity to perform activities and tasks that one normally expects of an adult (IOM, 1991).

Functional status: An individual's actual performance of activities and tasks associated with current life roles (IOM, 1991).

HITECH Act: The Health Information Technology for Economic and Clinical Health (HITECH) Act was enacted under Title XIII of the American Recovery and Reinvestment Act of 2009 and officially established the Office of the National Coordinator for Health Information Technology at the U.S. Department of Health and Human Services. The act includes incentives designed to accelerate the adoption of health information technology by the health care industry, health care providers, consumers, and patients, largely through the promotion of electronic health records and secure electronic exchange of health information.[3]

Internal validity: The extent to which a scientific study demonstrates a causal relation between two variables, satisfying the criteria of temporal precedence (the cause precedes the effect), covariation (cause and effect are related), and nonspuriousness (there is no plausible alternative explanation for the observed relationship) (Brewer, 2000).

Learning health care system: A health care system in which science, informatics, incentives, and culture are aligned for continuous improvement and innovation, with best practices being seamlessly embedded in the care process, patients and families being active participants in all elements of care, and new knowledge being captured as an integral by-product of the care experience (IOM, 2012).

Licensure: "The mandatory process by which a governmental agency grants time-limited permission to an individual to engage in a given occupation after verifying that he/she has met predetermined and standardized criteria and offers title protection for those who meet the criteria" (McHugh et al., 2014, p. 2; NOCA, 2005, p. 5).

---

[3] Health Information Technology for Economic and Clinical Health (HITECH) Act, Title XIII of Division A and Title IV of Division B of the American Recovery and Reinvestment Act of 2009 (ARRA), Public Law 111-5, 111th Congress, 1st session (February 17, 2009).

Manual: A psychotherapy treatment manual describes the theory, procedures, techniques, and strategies for a specific intervention and its indication. The procedures are detailed with scripts and case examples to define, illustrate, and operationalize the intervention. Manuals were developed to enhance internal validity and to reduce reliance on intuitive clinical judgment. They also ensure fidelity to the intended treatment and allow for rigorous replication by independent research groups. Following clinical trials, but sometimes before, manuals became books for dissemination of the psychotherapy, and many different adaptations were developed. Adaptations usually retained the core of the psychotherapy but were adapted for different age groups, cultures, formats of delivery, or disorders (Addis and Waltz, 2002; Fairburn and Cooper, 2011; Luborsky and DeRubeis, 1984).

Meaningful use: The use of certified electronic health record technology in a purposeful manner (such as electronic medication prescribing), ensuring that the technology is connected in a manner that provides for the electronic exchange of health information to improve the quality, cost, and outcomes of care (CDC, 2012; CMS, 2014).

Mechanism: How psychosocial interventions effect change, with causal links between treatment and outcomes (Kraemer, 2002).

Mediator: "In general, a given variable may be said to function as a mediator to the extent that it accounts for the relation between the predictor and the criterion. Mediators explain how external physical events take on internal psychological significance" (Baron and Kenny, 1986, p. 1176).

Meta-analysis: The process of using statistical methods to combine the results of similar studies quantitatively in an attempt to allow inferences to be drawn from the sample of studies and be applied to the population of interest (IOM, 2011).

Moderator: "In general terms, a moderator is a qualitative (e.g., sex, race, class) or quantitative (e.g., level of reward) variable that affects the direction and/or strength of the relation between an independent or predictor variable and a dependent or criterion variable" (Baron and Kenny, 1986, p. 1174).

MHPAEA: The Mental Health Parity and Addiction Equity Act (MHPAEA) is a federal law that requires group health plans and health insurance issuers to provide mental health or substance use (MH/SU) disorder benefits at levels equal to those of medical/surgical benefits.[4]

Patient-centered care: Health care that establishes a partnership among practitioners, patients, and their families (when appropriate) to ensure that decisions respect patients' wants, needs, and preferences and that patients have the education and support they need to make decisions and participate in their own care (IOM, 2001).

Patients: People with mental illnesses and/or chemical dependency who receive clinical care or treatment in medical settings where everyone with any type of condition (physical, mental, or emotional) is called a "patient."

Peer specialists: People with lived experience of mental illness and/or chemical dependency who act formally in roles that entail helping their peers to overcome and recover from mental illness and/or chemical dependency. They are also known as "peer mentors," "recovery support specialists," and "peer navigators."

Peer support: Services delivered by individuals who share life experiences with the people they are serving. These individuals offer informational, emotional, and intentional support to their peers, which allows for personal growth, wellness promotion, and recovery (SAMHSA, 2014).

Peers: People with mental illnesses and/or chemical dependency receiving services from peer specialists.

Pharmacotherapy: Therapy using pharmaceutical drugs.

Precision medicine: "An emerging approach for disease treatment and prevention that takes into account individual variability in genes, environment, and lifestyle for each person" (NIH, 2015).

Psychotherapy: "When a person speaks with a trained therapist in a safe and confidential environment to explore and understand feelings and behaviors and gain coping skills" (NAMI, 2015).

---

[4] Mental Health Parity and Addiction Equity Act (MHPAEA), amending section 712 of the Employee Retirement Income Security Act of 1974, section 2705 of the Public Health Service Act, and section 9812 of the Internal Revenue Code of 1986, H.R. 6983, 110th Congress, 2nd session (September 23, 2008).

Quality of evidence: "The extent to which one can be confident that the estimate of an intervention's effectiveness is correct" (IOM, 2011, p. 158).

Recovery: A process of change through which individuals improve their health and wellness, live a self-directed life, and strive to reach their full potential. The four major dimensions that support a life in recovery are overcoming or managing one's diseases or symptoms, having a stable and safe place to live, engaging in meaningful daily activities, and developing relationships and social networks (SAMHSA, 2010).

Registry: A data system developed for the purpose of collecting health-related information from special populations. Registries typically include all consumers with an illness, with no specified inclusion criteria, and collect data on any therapy used in any setting. Historically, registries have served as sources of information when no randomized controlled trial data are available. Registries are used to determine treatment safety and effectiveness, measure quality of care, and collect epidemiologic data.

Scientific rigor: Improves objectivity, minimizes bias, provides reproducible results, and fosters more complete reporting (IOM, 2011).

Standard: A process, action, or procedure that is deemed essential to producing scientifically valid, transparent, and reproducible results. A standard may be supported by scientific evidence, by a reasonable expectation that the standard helps achieve the anticipated level of quality, or by the broad acceptance of its practice (IOM, 2011).

Systematic review: A scientific investigation that focuses on a specific question and that uses explicit, planned scientific methods to identify, select, assess, and summarize the findings of similar but separate studies. It may or may not include a quantitative synthesis of the results from separate studies (i.e., meta-analysis) (IOM, 2011).

Systems-based approach: "An organized, deliberate approach to the identification, assessment, and management of a complex clinical problem; may include checklists, treatment algorithms, provider education, quality improvement initiatives, and changes in delivery and payment models" (Weissman and Meier, 2011, p. 2).

Vulnerable populations: "People from ethnic, cultural, and racial minorities, people with low educational attainment or low health literacy, and those in prisons or having limited access to care for geographic or financial reasons. Also included are people with serious illnesses, multiple chronic diseases, and disabilities (physical, mental, or cognitive), as well as those without access to needed health services" (IOM, 2015, p. 28).

REFERENCES

Addis, M. E., and J. Waltz. 2002. Implicit and untested assumptions about the role of psychotherapy treatment manuals in evidence-based mental health practice. *Clinical Psychology:
Science and Practice* 9(4):421-424.

Baron, R. M., and D. A. Kenny. 1986. The moderator-mediator variable distinction in social
psychological research: Conceptual, strategic, and statistical considerations. *Journal of
Personality and Social Psychology* 51:1173-1182.

The Bill & Melinda Gates Foundation. 2015. *Clinical trials.* https://docs.gatesfoundation.org/
documents/clinical_trials.pdf (accessed May 12, 2015).

Brewer, M. B. 2000. Research design and issues of validity. In *Handbook of research methods
in social and personality psychology,* edited by H. T. Reis and C. M. Judd. Cambridge,
MA: Cambridge University Press. Pp. 3-16.

CBO (Congressional Budget Office). 2013. *Dual-eligible beneficiaries of Medicare and Medicaid: Characteristics, health care spending, and evolving policies.* CBO publication no.
4374. Washington, DC: U.S. Government Printing Office.

CDC (Centers for Disease Control and Prevention). 2012. *Meaningful use: Introduction.*
http://www.cdc.gov/ehrmeaningfuluse/introduction.html (accessed May 8, 2015).

CMS (Centers for Medicare & Medicaid Services). 2014. *EHR incentive programs.* http://
www.cms.gov/RegulationsandGuidance/Legislation/HERIncentivePrograms/index.
html?redirect=/ehrincentiveprograms (accessed November 7, 2014).

_____. 2015. *The Mental Health Parity and Addiction Equity Act.* https://www.cms.gov/
CCIIO/Programs-and-Initiatives/Other-Insurance-Protections/mhpaea_factsheet.html (accessed June 23, 2015).

Fairburn, C. G., and Z. Cooper. 2011. Therapist competence, therapy quality, and therapist
training. *Behaviour Research and Therapy* 49(6):373-378.

Fink, A., J. Kosecoff, M. Chassin, and R. Brook. 1984. Consensus methods: Characteristics
and guidelines for use. *American Journal of Public Health* 74(9):979-983.

Hickey, J. V., L. Y. Unruh, R. P. Newhouse, M. Koithan, M. Johantgen, R. G. Hughes, K. B.
Haller, and V. A. Lundmark. 2014. Credentialing: The need for a national research
agenda. *Nursing Outlook* 62(2):119-127.

Holmboe, E. 2014. *Competency-based medical education (CBME) and transformation.* Pre-
sentation at the IOM's Future Directions of Credentialing Research in Nursing: A
Workshop, Washington, DC. http://www.iom.edu/~/media/Files/ActivityFiles/Workforce/
FutureDirectionsCNRworkshop/NCRWorkshopPresentations/DRAFT-EricHolmboe
FutureofNursingCredentialing.ppt (accessed December 18, 2014).

International Council of Nurses. 2009. *Credentialing: Fact sheet.* http://www.icn.ch/images/
stories/documents/publications/fact_sheets/1a_FS-Credentialing.pdf (accessed November
7, 2014).

IOM (Institute of Medicine). 1991. *Disability in America: Toward a national agenda for
prevention.* Washington, DC: National Academy Press.

_____. 2001. *Envisioning the national health care quality report.* Washington, DC: National
Academy Press.

_____. 2009. *Initial national priorities for comparative effectiveness research.* Washington,
DC: The National Academies Press.

_____. 2011. *Finding what works in health care: Standards for systematic reviews.* Washington, DC: The National Academies Press.

_____. 2012. *Best care at lower cost: The path to continuously learning health care in America.* Washington, DC: The National Academies Press.

_____. 2015. *Dying in America: Improving quality and honoring individual preferences near the end of life.* Washington, DC: The National Academies Press.

KFF (Kaiser Family Foundation). 2013. *Summary of the Affordable Care Act.* http://kff.org/health-reform/fact-sheet/summary-of-the-affordable-care-act (accessed May 19, 2015).

Kraemer, H. C. 2002. Mediators and moderators of treatment effects in randomized clinical trials. *Archives of General Psychiatry* 59(10):877-883.

Lauzon Clabo, L. 2014. *Core competencies in nursing credentialing and certification.* Presentation at the IOM's Future Directions of Credentialing Research in Nursing: A Workshop, Washington, DC. http://www.iom.edu/~/media/Files/ActivityFiles/Workforce/FutureDirectionsCNRworkshop/NCRWorkshopPresentations/3CoreCompetenciesinNursingCredentialingandCertificationpublicversion.pptx (accessed December 30, 2014).

Luborsky, L., and R. J. DeRubeis. 1984. The use of psychotherapy treatment manuals: A small revolution in psychotherapy research style. *Clinical Psychology Review* 4(1):5-14.

McHugh, M. D., R. E. Hawkins, P. E. Mazmanian, P. S. Romano, H. L. Smith, and J. Spetz. 2014. *Challenges and opportunities in nursing credentialing research design.* Discussion Paper, Institute of Medicine, Washington, DC. http://iom.edu/~/media/Files/Perspectives-Files/2014/Discussion-Papers/CredentientialingResearchDesign.pdf (accessed November 4, 2014).

NAMI (National Alliance on Mental Illness). 2015. *Psychotherapy.* https://www.nami.org/Learn-More/Treatment/Psychotherapy#sthash.kgOfTezP.dpuf (accessed May 8, 2015).

Needleman, J., R. S. Dittus, P. Pittman, J. Spetz, and R. Newhouse. 2014. *Nurse credentialing research frameworks and perspectives for assessing a research agenda.* Discussion Paper, Institute of Medicine, Washington, DC. http://www.iom.edu/~/media/Files/Perspectives-Files/2014/DiscussionPapers/CredentialingResearchFrameworks.pdf (accessed November 4, 2014).

Newhouse, R. 2014. *Understanding the landscape and state of science in credentialing research in nursing.* Presentation at the IOM's Future Directions of Credentialing Research in Nursing: A Workshop, Washington, DC. http://www.iom.edu/~/media/Files/ActivityFiles/Workforce/FutureDirectionsCNRworkshop/NCRWorkshopPresentations/Workshop_IOM_Newhouse.pdf (accessed December 18, 2014).

NIH (National Institutes of Health). 2015. *Precision medicine initiative.* http://www.nih.gov/precisionmedicine (accessed May 8, 2015).

NOCA (National Organization for Competency Assurance). 2005. *The NOCA guide to understanding credentialing concepts.* Washington, DC: NOCA.

Powell, C. 2003. The Delphi technique: Myths and realities. *Journal of Advanced Nursing* 41(4):376-382.

SAMHSA (Substance Abuse and Mental Health Services Administration). 2010. *SAMHSA's working definition of recovery: 10 guiding principles of recovery.* http://content.samhsa.gov/ext/item?uri=/samhsa/content/item/10007447/10007447.pdf (accessed May 8, 2015).

_____. 2014. *Peer support and social inclusion.* http://www.samhsa.gov/recovery/peer-support-social-inclusion (accessed May 8, 2015).

U.S. Department of Labor. 2014. *Credential resource guide.* http://wdr.doleta.gov/directives/attach/TEGL15-10a2.pdf (accessed November 7, 2014).

Weissman, D. E., and D. E. Meier. 2011. Identifying patients in need of a palliative care assessment in the hospital setting: A consensus report from the center to advance palliative care. *Journal of Palliative Medicine* 14(1):17-23.

Summary[1]

ABSTRACT

Approximately 20 percent of Americans are affected by mental health and substance use disorders, which are associated with significant morbidity and mortality. While the evidence base for the effectiveness of interventions to treat these disorders is sizable, a considerable gap exists between what is known to be effective and interventions that are actually delivered in clinical care. Addressing this quality chasm in mental health and substance use care is particularly critical given the recent passage of the Patient Protection and Affordable Care Act (ACA) and the Mental Health Parity and Addiction Equity Act, which are changing the delivery of care and access to treatments for mental health and substance use disorders. Increasing emphasis on accountability and performance measurement, moreover, will require strategies to promote and measure the quality of psychosocial interventions.

In this report, the study committee develops a framework that can be used to chart a path toward the ultimate goal of improving the outcomes of psychosocial interventions for those with mental health and substance use disorders. This framework identifies the key steps entailed in successfully bringing an evidence-based psychosocial intervention into clinical practice. It highlights the need

---

[1] This summary does not include references. Citations for the discussion presented in the summary appear in the subsequent report chapters.

to (1) support research to strengthen the evidence base on the efficacy and effectiveness of psychosocial interventions; (2) based on this evidence, identify the key elements that drive an intervention's effect; (3) conduct systematic reviews to inform clinical guidelines that incorporate these key elements; (4) using the findings of these systematic reviews, develop quality measures—measures of the structure, process, and outcomes of interventions; and (5) establish methods for successfully implementing and sustaining these interventions in regular practice, including the training of providers of these interventions. The committee intends for this framework to be an iterative one, with the results of the process being fed back into the evidence base and the cycle beginning anew. Central to the framework is the importance of using the consumer perspective to inform the process.

The recommendations offered in this report are intended to assist policy makers, health care organizations, and payers that are organizing and overseeing the provision of care for mental health and substance use disorders while navigating a new health care landscape. The recommendations also target providers, professional societies, funding agencies, consumers, and researchers, all of whom have a stake in ensuring that evidence-based, high-quality care is provided to individuals receiving mental health and substance use services.

Mental health and substance use disorders affect approximately 20 percent of Americans and are associated with significant morbidity and mortality. Although the current evidence base for the effects of psychosocial interventions is sizable, subsequent steps in the process of bringing a psychosocial intervention into routine clinical care are less well defined. The data from research supporting these interventions have not been well synthesized, and it can be difficult for consumers, providers, and payers to know what treatments are effective. This report details the reasons for the gap between what is known to be effective and current practice and offers recommendations for how best to address this gap by applying a framework that can be used to establish standards for psychosocial interventions.

Addressing the need for standards in mental health and substance use care is particularly critical given the recent passage of the Patient Protection and Affordable Care Act (ACA) and the Mental Health Parity and Addiction Equity Act. The ACA is aimed at reforming how care is delivered, with an emphasis on accountability and performance measurement, while the Mental Health Parity and Addiction Equity Act is intended to address limits on access to behavioral health care services. Without accepted and endorsed quality standards for psychosocial care, however, there may still be reluctance to promote appropriate use of these treatments. To counter pressures to limit access to psychosocial care, it is critical to promote the use of effective psychosocial interventions and to develop strategies for monitoring the quality of interventions provided.

In this context, the Institute of Medicine (IOM) convened an ad hoc committee to create a framework for establishing the evidence base for psychosocial interventions, and to describe the elements of effective interventions and the characteristics of effective service delivery systems.

STUDY CHARGE AND APPROACH

The American Psychiatric Association, American Psychological Association, Association for Behavioral Health and Wellness, National Association of Social Workers, National Institutes of Health, the Office of the Assistant Secretary for Planning and Evaluation within the U.S. Department of Health and Human Services, Substance Abuse and Mental Health Services Administration, U.S. Department of Veterans Affairs, asked the IOM to convene a committee to develop a framework for establishing standards for psychosocial interventions used to treat mental health and substance use disorders (see Box S-1 for the committee's full statement of task). Reflecting the complexity of this task, the 16-member committee comprised experts in a variety of disciplines, including psychiatry, psychology, social work, nursing, primary care, public health, and health policy. Members' areas of expertise encompassed clinical practice, quality and performance measurement, intervention development and evaluation, operation of health systems, implementation science, and professional education, as well as the perspectives of individuals who have been affected by mental health disorders. The scope of this study encompasses the full range of mental health and substance use disorders, age and demographic groups, and psychosocial interventions.

To complete its work, the committee convened for 5 meetings over the course of 12 months. It held public workshops in conjunction with two of these meetings to obtain additional information on specific aspects of the study charge (see Appendix A for further information).

KEY FINDINGS, CONCLUSIONS, AND RECOMMENDATIONS

The recommendations offered in this report are intended to assist policy makers, health care organizations, and payers that are organizing and overseeing the provision of care for mental health and substance use disorders while navigating a new health care landscape. The recommendations

BOX S-1
Statement of Task

The Institute of Medicine will establish an ad hoc committee that will develop a framework to establish efficacy standards for psychosocial interventions used to treat mental disorders. The committee will explore strategies that different stakeholders might take to help establish these standards for psychosocial treatments. Specifically, the committee will:

- Characterize the types of scientific evidence and processes needed to establish the effectiveness of psychosocial interventions.
  - Define levels of scientific evidence based on their rigor.
  - Define the types of studies needed to develop quality measures for monitoring quality of psychosocial therapies and their effectiveness.
  - Define the evidence needed to determine active treatment elements as well as their dose and duration.
- Using the best available evidence, identify the elements of psychosocial treatments that are most likely to improve a patient's mental health and can be tracked using quality measures. In addition, identify features of health care delivery systems involving psychosocial therapies that are most indicative of high-quality care that can be practically tracked as part of a system of quality measures. The following approaches to quality measurement should be considered:
  - Measures to determine if providers implement treatment in a manner that is consistent with evidence-based standards;
  - Measures that encourage continuity of treatment;
  - Measures that assess whether providers have the structures and processes in place to support effective psychotherapy;
  - Consumer-reported experiences of evidence-based psychosocial care; and
  - Consumer-reported outcomes using a measurement-based care approach.

also target providers, professional societies, funding agencies, consumers, and researchers, all of whom have a stake in ensuring that evidence-based, high-quality care is provided to individuals receiving mental health and substance use services. The committee's conclusions and recommendations are based on its review of the scientific evidence, information gathered in its public workshops, and the expert judgment of its members.[2] The commit-

---

[2] The committee's recommendations are numbered according to the chapter of the report in which they appear. Thus, for example, recommendation 2-1 is the first recommendation in Chapter 2. For purposes of clarity, some recommendations are presented in this summary in a different sequence from that in which they appear in the full report; however, their numeric designation remains the same.

tee offers recommendations for each component of its framework, which collectively offer a roadmap for implementing evidence-based psychosocial interventions.

Need for a Framework to Establish and Apply Efficacy Standards for Psychosocial Interventions

Mental health disorders encompass a range of conditions, including, for example, neurodevelopmental, anxiety, trauma, depressive, eating, personality, and psychotic disorders. Substance use disorders entail recurrent use of alcohol and legal or illegal drugs (e.g., cannabis, stimulants, hallucinogens, opioids) that cause significant impairment.

Mental health and substance use disorders are prevalent, affecting approximately 20 percent of the U.S. population. Moreover, the two categories of disorders are often comorbid, occurring together. The rate of comorbidity of mental, substance use, and physical disorders also is high. Approximately 18 percent of cancer patients, for example, have a comorbid mental health disorder. Comorbidity of any type leads to reduced compliance with medication, greater disability, and poorer chance of recovery. People with comorbid mental health, substance use, and physical disorders also are at increased risk of premature mortality from a variety of causes.

For purposes of this study, the committee defines psychosocial interventions for mental health and substance use disorders as *interpersonal or informational activities, techniques, or strategies that target biological, behavioral, cognitive, emotional, interpersonal, social, or environmental factors with the aim of reducing symptoms of these disorders and improving functioning or well-being.* These interventions include psychotherapies (e.g., psychodynamic therapy, cognitive-behavioral therapy, interpersonal psychotherapy, problem solving therapy), community-based treatments (e.g., assertive community treatment, first episode psychosis interventions), vocational rehabilitation, peer support services, and integrated care interventions. Interventions can be delivered in a variety of settings (e.g., outpatient clinics, individual provider offices, primary care clinics, schools, hospitals, community settings, and virtual settings such as telephone and video conferencing). Interventions occur in different formats (such as individual, family, group, computer-based) and can be administered by a variety of providers, from social workers, psychiatrists, and psychologists to religious leaders and peer providers. Psychosocial interventions can be stand-alone treatments or can be combined with other interventions, such as medication, for a range of disorders or problems. In addition, interventions can address psychosocial problems that negatively impact adherence to medical treatments or can deal with the interpersonal and social challenges present during recovery from a mental health or substance use problem. Sometimes multiple psychosocial interventions are employed.

The efficacy of a broad range of psychosocial interventions has been established through hundreds of randomized controlled clinical trials and numerous meta-analyses (described below). However, the quality of care that is actually delivered is less than ideal. Evidence-based psychosocial interventions often are not taught in programs training mental health and substance use providers and often are not available as part of routine clinical care for mental health and substance use disorders. This gap between what is known to be effective and the actual delivery of care is due to problems of access, insurance coverage, and fragmentation of care (different systems of providers, separation of primary and specialty care, different entities sponsoring and paying for care, and poor coordination of care, as well as variability in the training of numerous types of providers and the lack of requirements that evidence-based interventions be taught in training programs).

Over the course of its early meetings, it became clear to the committee that the development of the framework called for in its statement of task would be critical to charting a path toward the ultimate goal of improving the outcomes of psychosocial interventions for those with mental health and substance use disorders. In the context of developing this framework, the committee did not conduct a comprehensive literature review of efficacious interventions or systematically identify the evidence-based elements of interventions, but rather used the best of what is known about the establishment of an evidence-based intervention to build a framework that would make it possible to fully realize the high-quality implementation of evidence-based interventions in everyday care.

While this report addresses the types of studies needed to build an evidence base and the best methods for each phase of intervention development, testing, and dissemination, it does not create a compendium of study types and their respective rigor. Instead, it emphasizes via the framework the iterative nature of intervention science and the evolving methodologies that will be required to meet the psychosocial needs of individuals with mental health and substance use disorders. In this light, the committee does not define levels of scientific rigor in establishing an intervention as evidence based or specify the many interventions that have crossed the threshold for being identified as evidence based. Rather, the committee emphasizes an iterative framework that should guide the process of establishing the evidence base for psychosocial interventions and for the systems in which the interventions are delivered.

Key Findings

The information gathered for this study led to the following key findings concerning mental health and substance use disorders and the interventions developed to treat them:

- Mental health and substance use disorders are a serious public health problem.
- A wide variety of psychosocial interventions play a major role in the treatment of mental health and substance use disorders.
- Psychosocial interventions that have been demonstrated to be effective in research settings are not used routinely in clinical practice or taught in educational programs training mental health professionals who deliver psychosocial interventions.
- No standard system is in place to ensure that the psychosocial interventions delivered to patients/consumers are effective.

A Proposed Framework for Improving the Quality and Delivery of Psychosocial Interventions

Figure S-1 depicts the committee's framework, which identifies the key steps in successfully bringing an evidence-based psychosocial intervention into clinical practice. This framework highlights the need to

- support research to strengthen the evidence base on the efficacy and effectiveness of psychosocial interventions;
- based on this evidence, identify the key elements that drive the effects of an intervention;
- conduct systematic reviews to inform clinical guidelines that incorporate these key elements;
- using the findings of these systematic reviews, develop quality measures—measures of the structure, process, and outcomes of interventions; and
- establish methods for successfully implementing and sustaining these interventions in regular practice.

Central to this framework is the consumer perspective in informing the process. Evidence shows that consumers bring important perspectives and knowledge of mental health and substance use disorders. As applied to this framework, consumer involvement is important in identifying and formulating research questions for systematic review, helping to develop guideline recommendations, informing the development of quality measures, and monitoring the implementation of interventions. Consumer participation

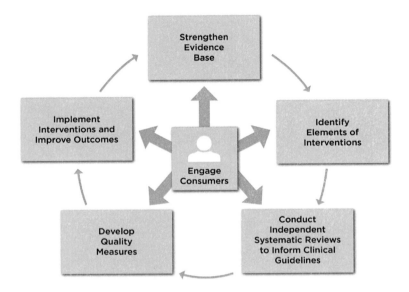

FIGURE S-1 Framework for developing standards for psychosocial interventions.

of this nature can lead to the development of interventions that address outcomes of importance to consumers, which in turn can lead to their increased participation in the interventions.

Importantly, the committee intends for the framework to be an iterative one, with the results of the process being fed back into the evidence base and the cycle beginning anew. Much has been done to establish the current evidence base for psychosocial interventions, but much more needs to be done to improve the quality of that evidence base; create new evidence-based interventions; engage consumers in this process; train the providers of psychosocial interventions; and ultimately streamline the process of developing, testing, implementing, and disseminating interventions that address the psychosocial needs of those with mental health and substance use problems.

The committee drew the following conclusions about the need for a framework:

> *The mental health and substance use care delivery system needs a framework for applying strategies to improve the evidence base for and increase the uptake of high-quality evidence-based interventions in the delivery of care.*

Broad stakeholder involvement is necessary to develop effective interventions that will lead to improved outcomes for individuals with mental health and substance use disorders.

Recommendation 2-1. *Use the committee's framework for improving patient outcomes through psychosocial interventions to strengthen the evidence base.* The U.S. Department of Health and Human Services should adopt the committee's framework to guide efforts to support policy, research, and implementation strategies designed to promote the use of evidence-based psychosocial interventions. Steps in this iterative process should focus on

- strengthening the evidence base for interventions,
- identifying key elements of interventions,
- conducting independent systematic reviews to inform clinical guidelines,
- developing quality measures for interventions, and
- implementing interventions and improving outcomes.

This is a complex process, and the framework is intended to be used to guide a continuous progression. At each step in the process, systematic research and evaluation approaches should be applied to iteratively expand the knowledge base for the development of new and improved standards for psychosocial interventions that will improve patient outcomes.

Recommendation 2-2. *Require consumer engagement.* The U.S. Department of Health and Human Services and other public and private funding agencies should ensure that consumers are active participants in the development of practice guidelines, quality measures, policies, and implementation strategies for, as well as research on, psychosocial interventions for people with mental health and substance use disorders, and provide appropriate incentives to that end. In addition, family members of consumers should be provided with opportunities to participate in such activities.

Strengthen the Evidence Base

The framework's cycle begins with strengthening the evidence base for identifying effective psychosocial interventions and their key elements. The data on these interventions are compelling. A number of meta-analyses have established the effects of psychosocial interventions on mental health and substance use disorders. Psychotherapies in particular have been subject to numerous meta-analyses. Few meta-analyses exist for other types of psychosocial interventions, such as suicide prevention programs, vocational rehabilitation, and clinical case management. However, these interventions have been subjected to randomized clinical trials and have been shown to have positive effects on the intended intervention target. Although meta-analyses support the use of psychosocial interventions in the treatment of mental health and substance use problems, additional studies are needed to further determine the utility of these interventions in different populations and settings, as well as to determine who is most capable of delivering the interventions, what the interventions' limitations are, and how best to implement them. Finally, there is a need to develop and test new interventions that are more effective and address currently unmet needs.

Identify Key Elements of Interventions

Once the evidence base for psychosocial interventions has been expanded, the next step is to identify the key elements that drive the effects of the interventions. Most evidence-based psychosocial interventions are standardized, and these standards are detailed in treatment manuals. Most if not all evidence-based, manualized psychosocial interventions are packages of multiple elements. An element is a therapeutic activity, technique, or strategy that is categorized as either "nonspecific"—fundamental, and occurring in most if not all psychosocial interventions (e.g., a trusting relationship with a therapist)—or "specific"—unique to a particular theoretical orientation and approach (e.g., systematic exposure to feared objects, a specific element of cognitive-behavioral therapy for anxiety). The application of effective interventions involves assembling combinations of elements that, based on evidence, are targeted to particular disorders and other patient characteristics The elements that make up evidence-based psychosocial interventions are clearly specified in measures of fidelity, which are used to ascertain whether a given intervention is implemented as intended in research studies, and to ensure that practitioners in training and practice are demonstrating competency in an intervention.

Furthermore, some elements identified as being specific are actually shared among certain manualized psychosocial interventions, although not always referred to with the same terminology, whereas others are unique. Recognition of the elements of evidence-based psychosocial interventions highlights their similarities as well as their true differences. However, this process of discovery is somewhat hampered by the lack of a common language for describing elements across different theoretical models and interventions. Examination of fidelity measures from different theoretical models indicates that different terms are used to describe the same element. For example, "using thought records" in cognitive-behavioral therapy is likely to represent the same element as "using mood ratings" in interpersonal psychotherapy. The field would benefit from a common terminology for identifying and classifying the elements across all evidence-based psychosocial interventions.

A common terminology for specific and nonspecific elements could offer several advantages for evidence-based psychosocial interventions. It would permit researchers to use the same terms so that data could be pooled from different research groups, resulting in a much larger database than can be achieved from independent studies of manualized interventions comprising multiple elements described using different terms. This database could be used to establish the optimal sequencing and dosing of elements and for whom a given element, or set of elements, is most effective. In addition, it might be possible to connect elements more precisely to purported mechanisms of change than is the case with an entire complex psychosocial intervention. In the future, an elements framework could advance training in and implementation of evidence-based psychosocial interventions, as practitioners would learn strategies and techniques that can be applied across target problems, disorders, or contexts.

Conduct Independent Systematic Reviews to Inform Clinical Guidelines

No national, standardized, and coordinated process exists in the United States for compiling, conducting, and disseminating systematic reviews, guidelines, and implementation materials for use by providers and by those formulating guidance for implementation and for insurance coverage. Since as far back as 1982, some in the field of mental health have suggested that a regulatory body be formed to conduct high-quality systematic reviews for psychosocial interventions, much as the U.S. Food and Drug Administration regulates all medications and most medical devices. It is this approval process that informs decisions on which medications and devices can be included for coverage by health plans and should be used by providers as effective interventions. While the concept of having a single entity oversee and approve the use of psychosocial interventions has practical appeal, it has not gained traction in the field and has not been supported by Congress. In an attempt to address this gap, professional organizations, health care organizations, federal entities, nonfederal organizations, and various researchers have independently reviewed the literature on psychosocial interventions. However, the result has been sets of guidelines that often are at odds with one another, and clinicians, consumers, providers, educators, and health care organizations seeking information are given little direction as to which reviews are accurate and which guidelines should be employed.

An important challenge in creating a standardized process for reviewing evidence is the fact that systematic reviews as currently conducted are laborious and costly, and rarely keep pace with advances in the field. To avoid the cost and timeliness problems inherent in systematic reviews, an entity charged with overseeing the reviews and their products could explore the potential for technology (e.g., the use of machine learning to augment and streamline the systematic review process) and clinical and research networks and learning environments to expedite the process and the development of updates to recommendations. In 2011, the IOM offered a set of recommendations for conducting high-quality systematic reviews. The guidelines broadly identify evidence-based treatments and approaches but generally are not designed to provide the level of detail needed to inform clinicians in the delivery of treatments to ensure reproducibility and a consistent level of quality outcomes. As a result, these guidelines would need to be modified to be more specific and ensure that information beyond intervention impact is available.

Having a process for systematically reviewing evidence is particularly important given the changes introduced under the ACA and the Mental Health Parity and Addiction Equity Act. Now more than ever, a standardized evaluation process is needed to enable the generation of reliable information to form the basis for policy and coverage decisions, curriculum development and training of clinicians, and other efforts to improve the quality of psychosocial care. Absent such a standardized process, the quality of care will continue to vary considerably. Systematic reviews need to address intervention efficacy, effectiveness, and implementation needs. Equally important is identifying the best information with which to answer these questions.

Two examples of the benefits of having a standardized, coordinated process for determining which interventions are evidence based are the National Institute for Health Care and Excellence (NICE) in the United Kingdom and the U.S. Department of Veterans Affairs' (VA's) Evidence-Based Synthesis Program (ESP). Both employ a coordinated process for conducting systematic reviews and creating guidelines based on internationally agreed-upon standards, and both have a process for evaluating the impact of guidelines on practice and outcomes. Based on the successes of NICE and the ESP, it is possible to develop a process for conducting systematic reviews and creating guidelines and implementation materials for psychosocial interventions, as well as a process for evaluating the impact of these tools, by leveraging existing resources.

The committee envisions a process that involves input from consumers and clinicians at every step. A potential direction is for the U.S. Department of Health and Human Services, in partnership with professional and consumer organizations, to develop a coordinated process for conducting systematic reviews of the evidence for psychosocial interventions and creating guidelines and implementation materials in accordance with the IOM standards for guideline development. Dissemination of practice guidelines and implementation tools resulting from the reviews could be conducted by the National Registry of Evidence-based Programs and Practices (NREPP) and professional organizations.

The committee drew the following conclusion about synthesizing evidence:

Approaches applied in other areas of health care (as recommended in previous IOM reports) can be applied in compiling and synthesizing evidence to guide care for mental health and substance use disorders.

Recommendation 4-1. *Expand and enhance processes for coordinating and conducting systematic reviews of psychosocial interventions and their elements.* The U.S. Department of Health and Human Services, in partnership with professional and consumer organizations, should expand and enhance existing efforts to support a coordinated process for conducting systematic reviews of psychosocial interventions and their elements based on the Institute of Medicine's recommendations for conducting high-quality systematic reviews. Research is needed to expedite the systematic review process through the use of machine learning and natural-language processing technologies to search databases for new developments.

Recommendation 4-2. *Develop a process for compiling and disseminating the results of systematic reviews along with guidelines and dissemination tools.* With input from the process outlined in Recommendation 4-1, the National Registry of Evidence-based Programs and Practices (NREPP) and professional organizations should disseminate guidelines, implementation tools, and methods for evaluating the impact of guidelines on practice and patient outcomes. This process should be informed by the models developed by the National Institute for Health Care and Excellence (NICE) in the United Kingdom and the U.S. Department of Veterans Affairs, and should be faithful to the Institute of Medicine standards for creating guidelines.

Develop Quality Measures

New care delivery systems and payment reforms being instituted under the ACA require measures for tracking the performance of the health care system. Quality measures are among the critical tools for health care providers and organizations during the process of transformation and improvement. To date, quality measures are lacking for key areas of mental health and substance use treatment. Of the 31 nationally endorsed measures related to these disorders, only 2 address a psychosocial intervention (screening and brief intervention for unhealthy alcohol use). This lack of measures reflects both limitations in the evidence base for determining what treatments are effective at achieving improvements in patient outcomes and challenges faced in obtaining from existing clinical data the detailed information necessary to support quality measurement.

To guide the consideration of opportunities to develop quality measures for psychosocial interventions, the committee built on prior work to offer an approach for the development of quality measures—structure, process, and outcome measures—for psychosocial interventions.

Structure measures are necessary to ensure that key elements of care can actually be implemented in a way that conforms to the evidence base linking those elements to key outcomes. Structure measures can be used to assess providers' training and capacity to offer evidence-based psychosocial interventions. They provide guidance on infrastructure development and best practices. They support credentialing and payment, thereby allowing purchasers and health plans both to select clinics or provider organizations that are equipped to furnish evidence-based psychosocial interventions and to provide incentives for the delivery of high-quality psychosocial care. They can support consumers in selecting providers with expertise in interventions specific to their condition or adapted to their cultural expectations. Finally, they can incorporate the capacity for the collection of outcome data.

Process measures are selected in areas where evidence from randomized controlled trials or observational studies has established an association between the provision of particular services in particular ways and the probability of achieving desired outcomes. The committee sees important opportunities to develop and apply process measures as part of a systematic, comprehensive, and balanced strategy for enhancing the quality of psychosocial interventions. While defining the processes of care associated with evidence-based psychosocial interventions is complicated, effective and efficient process measures provide important opportunities for the targeting and application of improvement strategies.

Of all quality measures, *outcome measures* have the greatest potential value for patients, families, clinicians, and payers because they indicate whether patients have improved or reached their highest level of function and whether full symptom or disease remission has been achieved. Importantly, outcome measures can be used to identify patients who are not responding to treatment or may require treatment modifications, to gauge individual provider and system performance, and to identify opportunities for quality improvement. Patient-reported outcomes are integral to measurement-based care, which is predicated on the use of brief, standardized, and specific assessment measures for target symptoms or behaviors that guide a patient-centered action plan.

Despite the diverse players in the quality field, there is a lack of strategic leadership and responsibility for the development and testing of quality measures for mental health and substance use care in general and for psychosocial interventions in particular. Furthermore, consumers have limited involvement in the development and implementation of quality measures in this arena. Systems for accountability and improvement need to focus on improving outcomes for individuals regardless of modality of treatment. However, the infrastructure for measurement and improvement of psychosocial interventions is lacking, both at the national level for measure development and at the local level for measure implementation and reporting. Current quality measures are insufficient to drive improvement in psychosocial interventions. While there is enthusiasm for incorporating performance measures based on patient-reported outcomes, there is no consensus on which outcomes should have priority and what tools are practical and feasible for use in guiding ongoing clinical care. In addition, risk adjustment methodologies need to be developed to ensure effective use of these measures for monitoring the performance of the health care system with respect to treatment for mental health and substance use disorders.

The committee drew the following conclusion about quality measurement for psychosocial interventions:

Approaches applied in other areas of health care can be applied in care for mental health and substance use disorders to develop reliable, valid, and feasible quality measures for both improvement and accountability purposes.

Recommendation 5-2. *Develop and continuously update a portfolio of measures with which to assess the structure, process, and outcomes of care.* The U.S. Department of Health and Human Services (HHS) should designate a locus of responsibility and leadership for the development of quality measures related to mental health and substance use disorders, with particular emphasis on filling the gaps in measures that address psychosocial interventions. HHS should support and promote the development of a balanced portfolio of measures for assessing the structure, process, and outcomes of care, giving priority to measuring access and outcomes and establishing structures that support the monitoring and improvement of access and outcomes.

Recommendation 5-3. *Support the use of health information technology for quality measurement and improvement of psychosocial interventions.* Federal, state, and private payers should support investments in the development of new and the improvement of existing data and coding systems to support quality measurement and improvement of psychosocial interventions. Specific efforts are needed to encourage broader use of health information technology and the development of data systems for tracking individuals' care and its outcomes over time and across settings. Registries used in other specialty care, such as bariatric treatment, could serve as a model. In addition, the U.S. Department of Health and Human Services should lead efforts involving organizations responsible for coding systems to improve standard code sets for electronic and administrative data (such as Current Procedural Terminology [CPT] and Systematized Nomenclature of Medicine [SNOMED]) to allow the capture of process and outcome data needed to evaluate mental health/substance use care in general and psychosocial interventions in particular. This effort will be facilitated by the identification of the elements of psychosocial interventions and development of a common terminology as proposed under Recommendation 3-1. Electronic and administrative data should include methods for coding disorder severity and other confounding and mitigating factors to enable the development and application of risk adjustment approaches, as well as methods for documenting the use of evidence-based treatment approaches.

Implement Interventions and Improve Outcomes

A comprehensive quality framework needs to consider properties beyond interventions themselves—in particular, the context in which interventions are delivered. This context includes characteristics of the consumer, the qualifications of the provider, the clinic or specific setting in which care is rendered, characteristics of the health system or organization in which the setting is embedded, and the regulatory and financial conditions under which the system or organization operates. Stakeholders in each of these areas can manipulate various levers that can shape the quality of the psychosocial interventions delivered to patients. Stakeholders and examples of levers as their disposal include

- consumers—meaningful participation in governance, in organizational leadership positions, and as board members;
- providers—quality measurement and reporting, such as tracking outcomes for practices and for populations served;
- provider organizations—electronic data systems with which to share medical records across disciplines and sites of service;
- health plans and purchasers—benefit design, such as pay-for-performance systems; and

- regulators—accreditation and licensure to help ensure the implementation of evidence-based practices.

Ignoring the context of an intervention and shortfalls in the manipulation of available levers can render a highly efficacious intervention unhelpful or even harmful. Growing evidence suggests that multifaceted implementation strategies targeting multiple levels of service provision—consumers, providers, organizations, payers, and regulators—are most effective. Much of the evidence surrounding the use of these levers to improve quality (in health care generally) is weak but promising, and should be augmented with further research.

The committee drew the following conclusion about improving the quality of psychosocial interventions:

Multiple stakeholders should apply levers, incentives, and other means to create learning health systems that continually progress toward higher quality (as recommended in previous IOM Quality Chasm reports).

Recommendation 6-1. *Adopt a system for quality improvement.* Purchasers, plans, and providers should adopt systems for measuring, monitoring, and improving quality for psychosocial interventions. These systems should be aligned across multiple levels. They should include structure, process, and outcome measures and a combination of financial and nonfinancial incentives to ensure accountability and encourage continuous quality improvement for providers and the organizations in which they practice. Quality improvement systems also should include measures of clinician core competencies in the delivery of evidence-based psychosocial interventions. Public reporting systems, provider profiling, pay-for-performance, and other accountability approaches that include outcome measures should account for differences in patient case mix (e.g., using risk adjustment methods) to counteract incentives for selection behavior on the part of clinicians and provider organizations, especially those operating under risk-based payment.

Recommendation 6-2. *Support quality improvement at multiple levels using multiple levers.* Purchasers, health care insurers, providers, consumers, and professional organizations should pursue strategies designed to support the implementation and continuous quality improvement of evidence-based psychosocial interventions at the provider, clinical organization, and health system levels.

- The infrastructure to support high-quality treatment includes ongoing provider training, consumer and family education, supervision, consultation, and leadership to enhance organizational culture and foster a climate for continuously learning health care systems. Other core aspects of infrastructure for the implementation and quality improvement of evidence-based psychosocial interventions include the use of registries, electronic health records, and computer-based decision support systems for providers and consumers, as well as technology-supported technical assistance and training.
- This infrastructure could be fostered by a nonprofit organization, supported and funded through a public–private partnership (e.g., the Institute for Healthcare Improvement), that would provide technical assistance to support provider organizations and clinicians in quality improvement efforts.

A Research Agenda

Additional research is needed to expand the evidence base on the effectiveness of psychosocial interventions, validate strategies for applying elements approaches, develop and test quality measures, and design and evaluate implementation strategies and policies. The committee offers the following recommendations as a research agenda to further progress in each phase of the framework.

Recommendation 3-1. *Conduct research to identify and validate elements of psychosocial interventions.* Public and private organizations should conduct research aimed at identifying and validating the elements of evidence-based psychosocial interventions across different populations (e.g., disorder/problem area, age, sex, race/ethnicity). The development and implementation of a research agenda is needed for

- developing a common terminology for describing and classifying the elements of evidence-based psychosocial interventions;
- evaluating the sequencing, dosing, moderators, mediators, and mechanisms of action of the elements of evidence-based psychosocial interventions; and
- continually updating the evidence base for elements and their efficacy.

Recommendation 4-3. *Conduct research to expand the evidence base for the effectiveness of psychosocial interventions.* The National Institutes of Health should coordinate research investments among federal, state, and private research funders, payers, and purchasers to develop and promote the adoption of evidence-based psychosocial interventions. This research should include

- randomized controlled trials to establish efficacy, complemented by other approaches encompassing field trials, observational studies, comparative effectiveness studies, data from learning environments and registries, and private-sector data;
- trials to establish the effectiveness of interventions and their elements in generalizable practice settings; and
- practice-based research networks that will provide "big data" to continuously inform the improvement and efficiency of interventions.

Recommendation 5-1. *Conduct research to contribute to the development, validation, and application of quality measures.* Federal, state, and private research funders and payers should establish a coordinated effort to invest in research to develop measures for assessing the structure, process, and outcomes of care, giving priority to

- measurement of access and outcomes;
- development and testing of quality measures, encompassing patient-reported outcomes in combination with clinical decision support and clinical workflow improvements;
- evaluation and improvement of the reliability and validity of measures;
- processes to capture key data that could be used for risk stratification or adjustment (e.g., severity, social support, housing);
- attention to documentation of treatment adjustment (e.g., what steps are taken when patients are not improving); and
- establishment of structures that support monitoring and improvement.

Recommendation 6-3. *Conduct research to design and evaluate strategies that can influence the quality of psychosocial interventions.* Research is needed to inform the design and evaluation of policies, organizational levers, and implementation/dissemination strategies that can improve the quality of psychosocial interventions and health outcomes. Potential supporters of this research include federal, state, and private entities.

- Policies should be assessed at the patient, provider, clinical organization/system, payer, purchaser, and population levels.

- Examples might include research to develop and assess the impact of benefit design changes and utilization management tools, new models of payment and delivery, systems for public reporting of quality information, and new approaches for training in psychosocial interventions.

CONCLUSION

The prevalence of mental health and substance use disorders and the impacts of these disorders on morbidity and mortality are well documented. The gap between what interventions are known to be effective and the care that is delivered, together with the changing landscape in health care, demands fundamental changes in processes used to ensure the availability and delivery of high-quality evidence-based psychosocial interventions. Determining the best ways to strengthen the evidence base, identify elements that underpin interventions, conduct systematic reviews to inform clinical guidelines, develop quality measures to track the effectiveness of interventions, and implement quality interventions to improve patient outcomes has been remarkably challenging for the field of mental health. The process of moving through each step of the committee's framework is complex, requires evidence, and should be iterative. The committee believes that its framework and its recommendations for action can help achieve the goal of improved outcomes from psychosocial interventions for individuals suffering from mental health and substance use disorders.

1

Introduction

Mental health and substance use disorders affect approximately 20 percent of Americans and are associated with significant morbidity and mortality. Substantial progress is needed to bring effective interventions to the treatment of those suffering from these disorders. Randomized controlled clinical trials have shown a wide range of psychosocial interventions to be efficacious in treating these disorders, but these interventions often are not being used in routine care. The gap between what is known to be effective and current practice has been defined as a "quality chasm" for health care in general (IOM, 2001) and for mental health and substance use disorders in particular (IOM, 2006). This report details the reasons for this quality chasm in psychosocial interventions for mental health and substance use disorders and offers recommendations for how best to address this chasm by applying a framework that can be used to establish standards for these interventions.

A variety of research approaches are available for establishing a psychosocial intervention as evidence based. Yet the subsequent steps entailed in bringing a psychosocial intervention into routine clinical care are less well defined. The current evidence base for the effects of psychosocial interventions is sizable, and includes thousands of studies on hundreds of interventions. Although many of these interventions have been found to be effective, the supporting data have not been well synthesized, and it can be difficult for consumers, providers, and payers to know what treatments are effective. In addition, implementation issues exist at the levels of providers, provider training programs, service delivery systems, and payers. In the

United States, moreover, there is a large pool of providers of psychosocial interventions, but their training and background vary widely. A number of training programs for providers of care for mental health and substance use disorders (e.g., programs in psychology and social work) do not require training in evidence-based psychosocial interventions, and in those that do require such training (e.g., programs in psychiatry), the means by which people are trained varies across training sites. Some programs provide a didactic in the intervention, while others employ extensive observation and case-based training (Sudak and Goldberg, 2012). Best strategies for updating the training of providers who are already in practice also are not well established. Furthermore, licensing boards do not require that providers demonstrate requisite skills in evidence-based practice (Isett et al., 2007). Even those providers who are trained may not deliver an intervention consistently, and methods for determining whether a provider is delivering an intervention as intended are limited (Bauer, 2002). It also is difficult to track an intervention to its intended outcome, as outcomes used in research are not often incorporated into clinical practice.

Finally, the availability of psychosocial interventions is highly influenced by the policies of payers. The levels of scientific evidence used to make coverage determinations and the types of studies and outcome measures used for this purpose vary widely. Payers currently lack the capacity to evaluate what intervention is being used and at what level of fidelity and quality, nor do they know how best to assess patient/client outcomes. As a result, it is difficult for consumers and payers to understand what they are buying.

Addressing the quality chasm at this time is particularly critical given the recent passage of the Patient Protection and Affordable Care Act (ACA) and the Mental Health Parity and Addiction Equity Act (MHPAEA).[1] The ACA is aimed at reforming how care is delivered, with an emphasis on accountability and performance measurement, while the MHPAEA is intended to address limits on access to behavioral health care services. Without accepted and endorsed quality standards for psychosocial care, however, there may still be reluctance to promote appropriate use of these treatments. To counter pressures to limit access to psychosocial care, it is critical to promote the use of effective psychosocial interventions and to develop strategies for monitoring the quality of interventions provided.

In this context, the Institute of Medicine (IOM) convened an ad hoc committee to create a framework for establishing the evidence base for

---

[1] Mental Health Parity and Addiction Equity Act (MHPAEA), amending section 712 of the Employee Retirement Income Security Act of 1974, section 2705 of the Public Health Service Act, and section 9812 of the Internal Revenue Code of 1986, Division C of Public Law 110-343, 110th Congress, 2nd session (October 3, 2008).

psychosocial interventions, and to describe the elements of effective interventions and the characteristics of effective service delivery systems.

STUDY CONTEXT

This study comes at a time of significant policy change. The enactment of the ACA is creating fundamental changes in the organization, financing, and delivery of health care. The act is intended to make care less fragmented, more efficient, and higher-quality through a number of provisions. Of particular relevance to the subject of this report, through the ACA, several million previously uninsured people have gained coverage for services to treat their mental health and substance use disorders. Health plans offered on the health insurance exchanges must include mental health and substance use services as essential benefits. One early model, developed prior to the ACA's full enactment, indicated that 3.7 million people with serious mental illness would gain coverage, as would an additional 1.15 million new users with less severe disorders (Garfield et al., 2011).[2]

In its broadest sense, the goal of the ACA is to achieve patient-centered, more affordable, and more effective health care. One prominent provision is a mandate for a National Quality Strategy,[3] which is focused on measuring performance, demonstrating "proof of value" provided by the care delivery system, exhibiting transparency of performance to payers and consumers, linking payment and other incentives/disincentives to performance, establishing provider accountability for the quality and cost of care, and reforming payment methodology (AHRQ, 2011). The National Quality Forum (NQF) was charged by the Centers for Medicare & Medicaid Services to compile, review, and endorse quality measures for use in gauging the quality and effectiveness of health care across many sectors of the health care system (CMS, 2014). Under certain provisions of the ACA, meeting the targets for these quality measures will serve as the basis for payment and for the application of other incentives/disincentives. Among those quality measures addressing mental health and substance use disorders, only two that focus on psychosocial interventions are NQF-endorsed.[4]

The ACA includes reforms with the potential to mitigate the division of mental health and substance use care between primary and specialty care. The act creates opportunities for large networks of providers to become accountable care organizations (ACOs)[5]—a care model that directly links

---

[2] This model assumed that Medicaid expansion would occur in all states, but because of a Supreme Court ruling in 2012, several states have opted out of Medicaid expansion.

[3] The National Quality Strategy is a strategic framework for policies designed to improve the quality of care by focusing on specific priorities and long-term goals.

[4] Brief alcohol screening and interventions.

[5] ACOs are large hospitals and/or physician groups.

care delivery, demonstration of quality, and cost-efficiency. The creation of ACOs will help drive the integration of mental health and substance use services into medical practice and vice versa.

The MHPAEA also has changed the health care landscape specifically for mental health and substance use disorders. The act requires that commercial health insurance plans and plans offered by employers with more than 50 employees that include mental health and substance use coverage place no day and visit limits on services for these disorders (as long as there are no such limits on medical services), and that cost-sharing provisions and annual maximums be set at the predominant level for medical services (HHS, 2013). In addition, MHPAEA regulations require parity for mental health/substance use and medical care in the application of care management techniques such as tiered formularies and utilization management tools. Whereas the MHPAEA deals only with group insurance offered by large employers with 51 or more employees, the ACA extends mental health and substance use coverage to plans offered by small employers and to individuals purchasing insurance through insurance exchanges. The ACA requires that benefit designs adhere to the provisions of the MHPAEA.

STUDY CHARGE AND APPROACH

The American Psychiatric Association, American Psychological Association, Association for Behavioral Health and Wellness, National Association of Social Workers, National Institutes of Health, the Office of the Assistant Secretary for Planning and Evaluation within the U.S. Department of Health and Human Services, Substance Abuse and Mental Health Services Administration, and the U.S. Department of Veterans Affairs asked the IOM to convene a committee to develop a framework for establishing standards for psychosocial interventions used to treat mental health and substance use disorders. The committee's full statement of task is presented in Box 1-1. Reflecting the complexity of this task, the 16-member committee included experts in a variety of disciplines, including psychiatry, psychology, social work, nursing, primary care, public health, and health policy. Members' areas of expertise encompassed clinical practice, quality and performance measurement, intervention development and evaluation, operation of health systems, implementation science, and professional education, as well as the perspectives of individuals who have been affected by mental health disorders. The scope of this study encompasses the full range of mental health and substance use disorders, age and demographic groups, and psychosocial interventions.

To complete its work, the committee convened for five meetings over the course of 12 months. It held public workshops in conjunction with two of these meetings to obtain additional information on specific aspects of

BOX 1-1
Statement of Task

The Institute of Medicine will establish an ad hoc committee that will develop a framework to establish efficacy standards for psychosocial interventions used to treat mental disorders. The committee will explore strategies that different stakeholders might take to help establish these standards for psychosocial treatments. Specifically, the committee will:

- Characterize the types of scientific evidence and processes needed to establish the effectiveness of psychosocial interventions.
  - Define levels of scientific evidence based on their rigor.
  - Define the types of studies needed to develop quality measures for monitoring quality of psychosocial therapies and their effectiveness.
  - Define the evidence needed to determine active treatment elements as well as their dose and duration.
- Using the best available evidence, identify the elements of psychosocial treatments that are most likely to improve a patient's mental health and can be tracked using quality measures. In addition, identify features of health care delivery systems involving psychosocial therapies that are most indicative of high-quality care that can be practically tracked as part of a system of quality measures. The following approaches to quality measurement should be considered:
  - Measures to determine if providers implement treatment in a manner that is consistent with evidence-based standards;
  - Measures that encourage continuity of treatment;
  - Measures that assess whether providers have the structures and processes in place to support effective psychotherapy;
  - Consumer-reported experiences of evidence-based psychosocial care; and
  - Consumer-reported outcomes using a measurement-based care approach.

the study charge (see Appendix A for further information). The committee's conclusions and recommendations are based on its review of the scientific evidence, information gathered in its public workshops, and the expert judgment of its members.

From the outset, it was clear to the committee that there is no generally accepted definition of psychosocial interventions in the literature. The committee offers a definition in this report that includes psychotherapies of various orientations for specific disorders (e.g., interpersonal, cognitive-behavioral, brief psychodynamic) and interventions that enhance outcomes across disorders (e.g., supported employment, supported housing, family psychoeducation, assertive community treatment, integrated programs for people with dual diagnoses, peer services).

The levels and quality of evidential support vary widely across the myriad psychosocial interventions. This variation reflects a reality in the field. The evidence base for some psychosocial interventions is extensive, while that for others, even some that are commonly used, is more limited. Given the committee's statement of task, the focus of this report is on evidence-based care, but this emphasis is not intended to discount the fact that many interventions may be effective but have not yet been established as evidence based. The long-term goal is for all psychosocial interventions to be grounded in evidence, and the intent of this study is to advance that goal.

To reflect the diversity in the field, the committee draws on evidence for a variety of approaches when possible. However, cognitive-behavioral therapy is discussed frequently in this report because it has been studied widely as an intervention for a number of mental health and substance use disorders and problems, tends to involve well-defined patient/client populations, has clearly described (i.e., manualized) intervention methods, is derived from a theoretical model, and has clearly defined outcomes. Other approaches have a less extensive evidence base.

In addressing its broad and complex charge, the committee focused on the need to develop a framework for establishing and applying efficacy standards for psychosocial interventions. Over the course of its early meetings, it became clear that the development of this framework would be critical to charting a path toward the ultimate goal of improving the outcomes of psychosocial interventions for those with mental health disorders; the committee also chose to make explicit the inclusion of substance use disorders. In the context of developing this framework, the committee did not conduct a comprehensive literature review of efficacious interventions[6] or systematically identify the evidence-based elements of interventions, but rather used the best of what is known about the establishment of an evidence-based intervention to build a framework that would make it possible to fully realize the high-quality implementation of evidence-based interventions in everyday care.

Importantly, the committee intends for the framework to be an iterative one, with the results of the process being fed back into the evidence base and the cycle beginning anew. Much has been done to establish the current

---

[6] Given the rigor and time involved in conducting a systematic review of the evidence for psychosocial interventions, this task is beyond the purview of the committee. Chapter 4 provides recommendations regarding how these systematic reviews should be conducted. This report also includes discussion of reviews conducted by the Agency for Healthcare Research and Quality, the Veterans Heath Administration, and the U.K. National Institute for Health and Care Excellence that meet the standards put forth in the IOM (2011) report *Finding What Works in Health Care: Standards for Systematic Reviews.*

evidence base for psychosocial interventions, but much more needs to be done to improve the quality of that evidence base; create new evidence-based interventions; actively engage consumers in this iterative process; train the providers of psychosocial interventions; and ultimately streamline the process of developing, testing, implementing, and disseminating interventions that address the psychosocial needs of those with mental health and substance use problems.

Perhaps the most straightforward aspect of the committee's charge was to define the levels of scientific evidence based on their rigor. From a simplistic point of view, the randomized controlled trial that compares an active intervention with a credible control condition is the gold standard, offering the best evidence that an intervention is efficacious. But the process of moving an intervention from development to testing for efficacy to effectiveness in the community and ultimately to dissemination requires a variety of different study types, all with their own standards for rigor. For example, the randomized controlled trial often is criticized because researchers enroll participants who may not resemble the people who may ultimately utilize the intervention. Thus studies that evaluate an intervention using real-world practicing clinicians and typical patient and client populations (e.g., effectiveness studies, field trials) increasingly are seen as generating valuable knowledge, although these studies vary in the extent to which traditional rigor is applied, based on the questions being addressed.

Also, more research is needed to understand what intervention is most effective for a given patient subgroup or individual. Emerging lines of research attempt to identify not just whether a specific intervention is effective but what pathway or sequence of intervention steps is most effective for specific clients or patients. Such studies have their own set of standards. Lastly, once an intervention becomes evidence based, it must be studied to determine how best to implement it in the real world, and to disseminate it to and ensure its quality implementation by providers. Such studies do not rely solely on the randomized controlled trial, as the question being addressed may best be answered using a different research method.

While this report addresses the study methods needed to build an evidence base and the best methods for each phase of intervention development, testing, and dissemination, the committee did not attempt to create a compendium of study types and their respective rigor. Rather, the framework is used to emphasize the iterative nature of intervention science and the evolving methodologies that will be required to address the psychosocial needs of individuals with mental health and substance use disorders. In this light, the committee does not define levels of scientific rigor in establishing an intervention as evidence based or specify the many interventions that have crossed the threshold for being identified as evidence based, but emphasizes that its iterative framework should guide the process of establishing the evidence base for psychosocial interventions and the systems in which those interventions are delivered.

The committee was charged "to identify the evidence needed to determine active treatment elements as well as their dose and duration." The effort to identify the active elements of psychosocial interventions has a long tradition in intervention development and research in the field of mental health and substance use disorders. Two perspectives emerge from this literature, focused on (1) the nature and quality of the interpersonal relationship between the interventionist and the client/patient, and (2) the content of the interchange between the interventionist and client/patient. Both of these perspectives have been demonstrated to be important components of evidence-based care. The charge to the committee thus requires that both of these traditions be included in its discussion of the active components of evidence-based interventions.

The recommendations offered in this report are intended to assist policy makers, health care organizations, and payers who are organizing and overseeing the provision of care for mental health and substance use disorders while navigating a new health care landscape. The recommendations also target providers, professional societies, funding agencies, consumers, and researchers, all of whom have a stake in ensuring that evidence-based, high-quality care is provided to individuals receiving mental health and substance use services.

OVERVIEW OF MENTAL HEALTH AND SUBSTANCE USE DISORDERS: PREVALENCE, DISABLING EFFECTS, AND COSTS

Mental health disorders encompass a range of conditions, including, for example, neurodevelopmental, anxiety, trauma, depressive, eating, personality, and psychotic disorders. Substance use disorders encompass recurrent use of alcohol and legal or illegal drugs (e.g., cannabis, stimulants, hallucinogens, opioids) that cause significant impairment.

Mental health and substance use disorders are prevalent and highly disabling. The 2009-2010 National Surveys on Drug Use and Health, for example, found that approximately 20 percent of the U.S. population had experienced a mental disorder in the past year and 8.9 percent a substance use disorder (SAMHSA, 2012b). The two often are comorbid, occurring together (Drake and Mueser, 2000). Studies have found that 15 percent of those with a mental disorder in a given year also have a substance use disorder, and 60 percent of those with a substance use disorder in a given year also have a mental disorder (HHS, 1999). The rate of comorbidity of mental, substance use, and physical disorders also is high; approximately 18 percent of cancer patients, for example, have a comorbid mental disorder (Nakash et al., 2014). Comorbidity of any type leads to reduced compliance with medication, greater disability, and a poorer chance of recovery (Drake and Mueser, 2000). Among diabetics, for example, comorbid depression adversely affects adherence to diet and exercise regimens and smoking cessation, as well as adherence to medications for diabetes, hypertension, and hyperlipidemia (Lin et al., 2004). People with comorbid mental health, substance use, and physical disorders also are at increased risk of premature mortality from a variety of causes (Katon et al., 2008; Thomson, 2011), perhaps because mental health and substance use disorders complicate the management of comorbid chronic medical conditions (Grenard et al., 2011). Depression after a heart attack, for example, roughly triples the risk of dying from a future heart attack, according to multiple studies (Bush et al., 2005).

The World Health Organization's (WHO's) Global Burden of Disease Study 2010 evaluates disability across all major causes of disease in 183 countries, using disability-adjusted life-years (DALYs)[7] (Whiteford et al., 2013). Findings indicate that mental health and substance use disorders accounted for 7.4 percent of all DALYs and ranked fifth among 10 categories of disease. Further, they ranked first worldwide in years lost to disability, at 22.9 percent (see Table 1-1). Among mental health and substance use disorders, depression was the most disabling, accounting for 40.5 percent of DALYs. Ranking below depression were anxiety disorders (14.6 percent), illicit drug use disorders (10.9 percent), alcohol use disorders (9.6 percent), schizophrenia (7.4 percent), bipolar disorder (7.0 percent), pervasive developmental disorders (4.2 percent), childhood behavioral disorders (3.4 percent), and eating disorders (1.2 percent).

Mental health and substance disorders impose high direct costs for care, as well as indirect costs (Kessler, 2012). It is estimated that in 2005, care for these disorders in the United States cost a total of $135 billion (Mark et al., 2011). They also imposed indirect costs due to reduced productivity in the workplace in the form of absenteeism, "presenteeism" (i.e., attending work with symptoms impairing performance), days of disability, and workplace accidents. Furthermore, mental health and substance use disorders are responsible for decreased achievement by children in school and an increased burden on the child welfare system. These disorders also impose a high burden on the juvenile justice system: fully 60-75 percent of young people in the juvenile justice system have a mental disorder (Teplin et al., 2002). Likewise, approximately 56 percent of state prisoners, 45 percent of federal prisoners, and 64 percent of jail inmates have a mental disorder (BJS, 2006). The rate of substance use disorders, many of which are comor-

---

[7] DALYs denote the number of years of life lost due to ill health; disability; or early death, including suicide. A DALY represents the sum of years lost to disability (YLDs) and years of life lost (YLLs).

TABLE 1-1 Leading Causes of Disease Burden

Condition	Proportion of Total DALYs (95% UI)	Proportion of Total YLDs (95% UI)	Proportion of Total YLLs (95% UI)
Cardiovascular and circulatory diseases	11.9% (11.0-12.6)	2.8% (2.4-3.4)	15.9% (15.0-16.8)
Diarrhea, lower respiratory infections, meningitis, and other common infectious diseases	11.4% (10.3-12.7)	2.6% (2.0-3.2)	15.4% (14.0-17.1)
Neonatal disorders	8.1% (7.3-9.0)	1.2% (1.0-1.5)	11.2% (10.2-12.4)
Cancer	7.6% (7.0-8.2)	0.6% (0.5-0.7)	10.7% (10.0-11.4)
Mental and substance use disorders	7.4% (6.2-8.6)	22.9% (18.6-27.2)	0.5% (0.4-0.7)
Musculoskeletal disorders	6.8% (5.4-8.2)	21.3% (17.7-24.9)	0.2% (0.2-0.3)
HIV/AIDS and tuberculosis	5.3% (4.8-5.7)	1.4% (1.0-1.9)	7.0% (6.4-7.5)
Other noncommunicable diseases	5.1% (4.1-6.6)	11.1% (8.2-15.2)	2.4% (2.0-2.8)
Diabetes and urogenital, blood, and endocrine diseases	4.9% (4.4-5.5)	7.3% (6.1-8.7)	3.8% (3.4-4.3)
Unintentional injuries other than transport injuries	4.8% (4.4-5.3)	3.4% (2.5-4.4)	5.5% (4.9-5.9)

NOTE: DALYs = disability-adjusted life-years; UI = uncertainty interval; YLDs = years lived with a disability; YLLs = years of life lost.
SOURCE: Whiteford et al., 2013.

bid with mental disorders, is similarly high among prison inmates (Peters et al., 1998). Still, only 39 percent of the 45.9 million adults with mental disorders used mental health services in 2010 (SAMHSA, 2012a). And according to the National Comorbidity Survey Replication, conducted in 2001-2003, a similarly low percentage of adults with comorbid substance use disorders used services (Wang et al., 2005). States bear a large proportion of the indirect costs of mental health and substance disorders through their disability, education, child welfare, social services, and criminal and juvenile justice systems.

PSYCHOSOCIAL INTERVENTIONS

Definition

To guide our definition of psychosocial interventions, the committee built on the approach to defining interventions used in the Consolidated Standards of Reporting Trials for Social and Psychological Interventions (CONSORT-SPI; Grant, 2014).[8]

The term "intervention" means "the act or . . . a method of interfering with the outcome or course especially of a condition or process (as to prevent harm or improve functioning)" (*Merriam-Webster Dictionary*) or "acting to intentionally interfere with an affair so to affect its course or issue" (*Oxford English Dictionary*). These definitions emphasize two constructs—an *action* and an *outcome*. Psychosocial interventions capitalize on psychological or social actions to produce change in psychological, social, biological, and/or functional outcomes. CONSORT-SPI emphasizes the construct of *mediators*, or the ways in which the action leads to an outcome, as a way of distinguishing psychosocial from other interventions, such as medical interventions (Montgomery et al., 2013). Based on these sources, modified for mental health and substance use disorders, the committee proposes the following definition of psychosocial interventions:

> *Psychosocial interventions for mental health and substance use disorders are interpersonal or informational activities, techniques, or strategies that target biological, behavioral, cognitive, emotional, interpersonal, social, or environmental factors with the aim of improving health functioning and well-being.*

This definition, illustrated in Figure 1-1, incorporates three main concepts: action, mediators, and outcomes. The action is defined as *activities, techniques, or strategies* that are delivered interpersonally (i.e., a relation-

---

[8] This text has been updated since the prepublication version of this report.

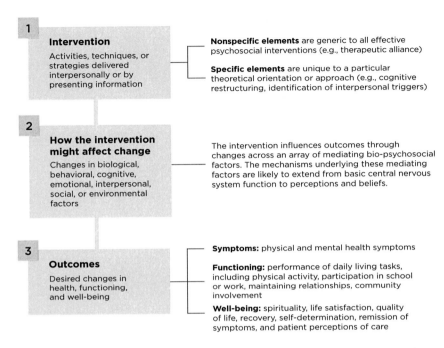

FIGURE 1-1 Illustration of the three main concepts in the committee's definition of psychosocial interventions.

ship between a practitioner and a client) or through the presentation of information (e.g., bibliotherapy, Internet-based therapies, biofeedback). The activities, techniques, or strategies are of two types: (1) nonspecific elements that are common to all effective psychosocial interventions, such as the therapeutic alliance, therapist empathy, and the client's hopes and expectations; and (2) specific elements that are tied to a particular theoretical model or psychosocial approach (e.g., communication skills training, exposure tasks for anxiety).

Mediators are the ways in which the action of psychosocial interventions leads to a specific outcome through *changes in biological, behavioral, cognitive, emotional, interpersonal, social, or environmental factors*; these changes explain or mediate the outcome. Notably, these changes are likely to exert their effects through an array of mechanisms in leading to an outcome (Kraemer et al., 2002), and can extend from basic central nervous system function to perceptions and beliefs.

Finally, outcomes of psychosocial interventions encompass desired changes in three areas: (1) *symptoms*, including both physical and mental

health symptoms; (2) *functioning*, or the performance of activities, including but not limited to physical activity, activities of daily living, assigned
tasks in school and work, maintaining intimate and peer relationships, rais-
ing a family, and involvement in community activities; and (3) *well-being*,
including spirituality, life satisfaction, quality of life, and the promotion
of recovery so that individuals "live a self-directed life, and strive to reach
their full potential" (SAMHSA, 2012a). Psychosocial interventions have
broader societal outcomes as well, such as utilization of acute or institutional services and disability costs. However, these outcomes are not the
direct focus of the intervention and therefore are not included in the definition here.

Application of Psychosocial Interventions

The committee's definition of psychosocial interventions is applicable
across a wide array of settings, formats, providers, and populations.

Settings and Formats

The broad range of settings in which psychosocial interventions are delivered includes outpatient clinics, solo provider offices, primary care clinics, schools, client homes, hospitals and other facilities (including inpatient
and partial hospital care), and community settings (e.g., senior services,
religious services). Some interventions use a combination of office-based
and naturalistic sites, and some are designed for specific environments.

While historically, most psychosocial interventions have been delivered
in an interpersonal format with face-to-face contact between provider and
client, recent real-time delivery formats include telephone, digital devices,
and video conferencing, all of which are called "synchronous" delivery.
There are also "asynchronous" delivery formats that include self-guided
books (bibliotherapy) and computer/Internet or video delivery, with minimal face-to-face contact between provider and client. Some interventions
combine one or more of these options. Formats for psychosocial interventions also include individual, family, group, or milieu, with varying intensity
(length of sessions), frequency (how often in a specified time), and duration
(length of treatment episode).

Providers

Providers who deliver psychosocial interventions include psychologists,
psychiatrists, social workers, counselors/therapists, primary care and other
nonpsychiatric physicians, nurses, physical and occupational therapists,
religious leaders, lay and peer providers, paraprofessionals and caregiv-

ers, and automated providers (e.g., Internet/audio/video-delivered interventions). Combinations of provider options are sometimes used.

Populations

The population targeted by psychosocial interventions is varied. It includes individuals at risk of or experiencing prodromal symptoms of an illness; individuals with acute disorders; individuals in remission, maintenance, or recovery phases of disorders; and individuals who are not ill but are challenged by daily functioning, relationship problems, life events, or psychological adjustment.

Examples of Psychosocial Interventions

There is no widely accepted categorization of psychosocial interventions. The term is generally applied to a broad range of types of interventions, which include psychotherapies (e.g., psychodynamic therapy, cognitive-behavioral therapy, interpersonal psychotherapy, problem solving therapy), community-based treatment (e.g., assertive community treatment, first episode psychosis interventions); vocational rehabilitation, peer support services, and integrated care interventions. The full list, which is too long to reproduce here, consists of interventions from a wide range of theoretical orientations (e.g., psychodynamic, behavioral, social justice, attachment, recovery, and strength-based theories). Each theoretical orientation encompasses a variety of interventions (e.g., within psychodynamic orientations are relational versus ego psychological approaches; within behavioral orientations are cognitive and contingency management approaches). (See Box 1-2 for three examples.)

Efficacy of Psychosocial Interventions

The efficacy of a broad range of psychosocial interventions has been established through hundreds of randomized controlled clinical trials and numerous meta-analyses (Barth et al., 2013; Cuijpers et al., 2010a,b, 2011, 2013; IOM, 2006, 2010). See Chapter 2 for further discussion of evidence-based psychosocial interventions.

Psychosocial interventions often are valuable on their own but also can be combined with other interventions, such as medication, for a range of disorders or problems. In addition, interventions can address psychosocial problems that negatively impact adherence to medical treatments or can deal with the interpersonal and social challenges present during recovery from a mental health or substance use problem. Sometimes multiple psychosocial interventions are employed.

BOX 1-2
Examples of Psychosocial Interventions

Assertive community treatment encompasses an array of services and interventions provided by a community-based, interdisciplinary, mobile treatment team (Stein and Test, 1980). The team consists of case managers, peer support workers, psychiatrists, social workers, psychologists, nurses, and vocational specialists. The approach is designed to provide comprehensive, community-based psychiatric treatment, rehabilitation, and support to persons with serious mental health and substance use disorders, such as bipolar disorder and schizophrenia. A fundamental goal is to provide supports and help consumers develop skills so they can maintain community living, avoid hospitalization, improve their quality of life, and strive for recovery. The core features of assertive community treatment are individualization and flexibility of services based on recovery goals; small caseloads; assertive outreach; ongoing treatment and support, including medication; and 24-hour availability with crisis readiness and a range of psychosocial interventions, such as family psychoeducation, supported employment, dual-disorder substance abuse treatment, and motivational interviewing.

Cognitive-behavioral therapy is used for a wide array of mental health and substance use disorders. It combines behavioral techniques with cognitive psychology—the scientific study of mental processes, such as perception, memory, reasoning, decision making, and problem solving. The goal is to replace maladaptive behavior and faulty cognitions with thoughts and self-statements that promote adaptive behavior (Beck et al., 1979). One example is to replace a defeatist expectation, such as "I can't do anything right," with a positive expectation, such as "I can do this right." Therapy focuses primarily on the "here and now" and imparts a directive or guidance role to the therapist, a structuring of the psychotherapy sessions, and the alleviation of symptoms and patients' vulnerabilities. Some of the elements of cognitive-behavioral therapy include cognitive restructuring, exposure techniques, behavioral activation, relaxation training, self-monitoring, and relapse prevention.

Contingency management is a psychosocial intervention designed for substance use disorders. As an evidence-based practice based on operant conditioning principles, it uses an incentive-based approach that rewards a client contingent upon meeting desired outcomes. Incentives found to be effective include both voucher/cash equivalents (guaranteed payment) and "prize-based" approaches that feature the chance to earn a large prize, while most chances are low value (Higgins and Silverman, 2008; Stitzer and Petry, 2006).

Not only are psychosocial interventions effective, but patients/clients often prefer them to medications for mental health and substance use disorders when the two approaches have similar efficacy. A recent meta-analysis of 34 studies encompassing 90,483 participants found a threefold higher preference for psychotherapy (McHugh et al., 2013): 75 percent of patients, especially younger patients and women, preferred psychotherapy. Interventions also can be important to provide an alternative for those for whom medication treatment is inadvisable (e.g., pregnant women, very young children, those with complex medical conditions); to enhance medication compliance, or to deal with the social and interpersonal issues that complicate recovery from mental health and substance use disorders.

Despite patients' preference for psychosocial interventions, a recent review of national practice patterns shows a decline in psychotherapy and an increase in use of antidepressants (Cherry et al., 2007). From 1998 to 2007, receipt of "psychotherapy only" declined from 15 percent to 10.9 percent of those receiving outpatient mental health care, whereas use of "psychotropic medication only" increased from 44.1 percent to 57.4 percent. The use of combination treatment—both psychotherapy and psychotropic medication—decreased from 40 percent to 32.1 percent (Marcus and Olfson, 2010).

QUALITY CHALLENGES AND THE NEED
FOR A NEW FRAMEWORK

The Quality Problem

Quality of care refers to "the degree to which health services for individuals and populations increase the likelihood of desired health outcomes and are consistent with current professional knowledge" (IOM, 1990, p. 21). An IOM committee evaluating mental health counseling services (IOM, 2010) concluded that high-quality care is achieved through a patient-centered system of quality measurement, monitoring, and improvement grounded in evidence.

The quality of care for both physical and mental health and substance use disorders is less than ideal. In a study of 13,275 individuals, researchers from the RAND Corporation searched for quality indicators in medical records (McGlynn et al., 2003). Overall, among patients with a wide array of physical and mental disorders, only 54.9 percent had received recommended care. The nationally representative National Comorbidity Survey Replication found that only 32.7 percent of patients had received at least minimally adequate treatment, based on such process measures as a low number of psychotherapy sessions and medication management visits (Wang et al., 2005). Likewise, only 27 percent of the studies included in a large review of studies published from 1992 to 2000 reported adequate rates of adherence to mental health clinical practice guidelines (Bauer, 2002). In a series of reports, the IOM (1999, 2001, 2006) has called attention to the quality problem: a 2006 IOM report on quality of care for mental health and substance use conditions found that a broad range of evidence-based psychosocial interventions were not being delivered in routine practice. This problem is especially widespread in primary care, where mental health and substance use disorders often go undetected, untreated, or poorly treated (Mitchell et al., 2009; Wood et al., 2013; Young et al., 2001).

Reasons for the Quality Problem

Some large national organizations (e.g., the U.S. Department of Veterans Affairs [VA] health care system [Karlin and Cross, 2014]) have developed their own programs to ensure that evidence-based psychosocial interventions are available in routine care. In general, however, evidence-based psychosocial interventions often are not available as part of routine clinical care for mental health and substance use disorders (IOM, 2006). The fragmentation of care for these disorders is one of the reasons for the quality chasm. Care is characterized by different systems of specialty providers; separation of primary and specialty care; and different state and federal agencies—including health, education, housing, and criminal justice—sponsoring or paying for care. Poor coordination of care can result in unnecessary suffering, excess disability, and earlier death from treatable conditions tied to modifiable risk factors, such as obesity, smoking, substance use, and inadequate medical care (Colton and Manderscheid, 2006).

Fragmentation also occurs in training, with specialty providers being trained in medical schools and in psychology, social work, nursing, and counseling programs. One large survey of a random sample of training directors from accredited training programs in psychiatry, psychology, and social work found that few programs required both didactic and clinical supervision in any evidence-based psychotherapy (Weissman et al., 2006). While a follow-up study has not been published, new developments suggest some improvements. The American Psychiatric Association now urges that evidence of competence in psychodynamic therapy, cognitive-behavioral therapy, brief treatment, and combined treatment with medication be collected in residency training. In its new accreditation standards, still in the public comment stage, the American Psychological Association calls on doctoral training programs to focus on "integration of empirical evidence and practice" (APA, 2015). And the 2008 accreditation standards of the Council on Social Work Education require that social work trainees "employ evidence-based interventions" (CSWE, 2008). Despite these positive steps, however, training programs are given little guidance as to which practices are evidence based, what models of training are most effective, or how the acquisition of core competencies should be assessed (see the full discussion in Chapter 6).

Potential Solutions to the Quality Problem

Potential solutions to the quality problem include identifying the elements of therapeutic change, establishing a coordinated process for reviewing the evidence, creating credentialing standards, and measuring quality of care.

Identifying Elements of Therapeutic Change

For some disorders, such as depression, there are a variety of psychosocial interventions from varying theoretical orientations; for other disorders, such as posttraumatic stress disorder, there are multiple manualized interventions derived from the same theoretical model. Moreover, a number of interventions are adaptations of other interventions targeting different ages, delivery methods (e.g., individual, group), or settings (e.g., primary care, private practice). Considering that most interventions comprise various therapeutic activities, techniques, or strategies (hereafter called "elements")—some of which are shared across different interventions, even across different theoretical orientations, and some of which are unique to given interventions—the committee recognized the potential value of developing a common terminology for the elements of psychosocial interventions.[9] Among other advantages, having such a terminology could facilitate optimally matching the elements of evidence-based interventions to the needs of the individual patient.

In addition to better enabling an understanding of how psychosocial interventions work, the concept of identifying elements has the advantage of making treatments more accessible. Uncovering therapeutic elements that cut across existing interventions and address therapeutic targets across disorders and consumer populations may allow psychosocial interventions to become far more streamlined and easier to teach to clinicians, and potentially make it possible to provide rapid intervention for consumers. The committee also acknowledges the challenges associated with this approach. For example, some interventions may not lend themselves well to an elements approach.

---

[9] Although this report uses the more familiar word "terminology," the committee recognizes that the term "ontology" may be helpful in that it describes an added dimension of interconnectedness among elements, beyond simply defining them. This is supported by the IOM (2014) report *Capturing Social and Behavioral Domains and Measures in Electronic Health Records: Phase 2.*

Establishing a Coordinated Process for Reviewing the Evidence

Building of the evidence base for an elements approach will not occur overnight, and the committee anticipates many years of development before even a few therapeutic elements have been identified. Additionally, methods will be needed for ensuring that those credentialed to deliver an elements approach continue to use the skills in which they are trained. One way to expedite efforts to solve the quality problem would be to identify a process by which evidence on psychosocial interventions could be reviewed objectively using a predetermined set of review standards and the evidence base updated in a reasonable timeframe to reflect the most recent advances in the field. This process would also allow for addressing situations in which evidence is limited and considering different sources of data when the scientific evidence is lacking. Finally, the process would need to be coordinated and organized so as to limit confusion about just what is evidence based. Currently, systematic reviews and guidelines are created by different organizations, using different review standards, and the result can be conflicting information. Having a coordinated body to set the standards and review the evidence base would mitigate this confusion.

Creating Credentialing Standards

Another solution to the quality chasm is to create an agreed-upon set of credentialing standards to ensure that providers are trained to deliver evidence-based practices. As has been the case in the VA and in the United Kingdom's National Health Service, creating a credentialing process to ensure that providers can deliver evidence-based psychosocial interventions and their elements will require that people and organizations involved in the credentialing process engage in a dialogue to determine what core competencies providers need to provide high-quality interventions, what training practices can best ensure that providers are supported to learn these practices, and whether providers need to be recredentialed periodically. Additionally, research is sorely needed to determine which training practices are effective. Many training practices in current use have not undergone rigorous evaluation, and some practices that are known to be effective (e.g., videotape review of counseling sessions by experts) are expensive and difficult to sustain.

Measuring Quality of Care

The committee determined that it will be necessary to develop measures of quality care for psychosocial interventions to ensure that consumers are receiving the best possible treatment (see Chapter 5). Research to develop quality measures from electronic health records is one potential means of improving how quality is determined. Research is needed as well to identify practice patterns associated with performance quality. A systematic way to review quality also needs to be established.

KEY FINDINGS

The committee identified the following key findings about mental health and substance use disorders and the interventions developed to treat them:

- Mental health and substance use disorders are a serious public health problem.
- A wide variety of psychosocial interventions play a major role in the treatment of mental health and substance use conditions.
- Psychosocial interventions that have been demonstrated to be effective in research settings are not used routinely in clinical practice.
- No standard system is in place to ensure that the psychosocial interventions delivered to patients/consumers are effective.

ORGANIZATION OF THE REPORT

This report is organized into six chapters. Chapter 2 presents the committee's framework for applying and strengthening the evidence base for psychosocial interventions. The remaining chapters address in turn the steps in this framework. Chapter 3 examines the elements of therapeutic change that are common to a myriad of psychosocial interventions; the identification and standardization of these elements is the first essential step in strengthening the evidence base for psychosocial interventions. Chapter 4 addresses the standards, processes, and content for the independent evidence reviews needed to inform clinical guidelines. Chapter 5 looks at the development of measures for the quality of care for mental health and substance use disorders. Finally, Chapter 6 explores the levers available to the various stakeholders for improving the outcomes and quality of care. The committee's recommendations are located at the end of each of these chapters. Table 1-2 shows the chapters in which each component of the committee's statement of task (see Box 1-1) is addressed.

TABLE 1-2 Elements of the Statement of Task and Chapters Where They Are Addressed

Element of the Statement of Task	Chapters
The Institute of Medicine will establish an ad hoc committee that will develop a framework to establish efficacy standards for psychosocial interventions used to treat mental disorders. The committee will explore strategies that different stakeholders might take to help establish these standards for psychosocial treatments.	Chapter 2: A Proposed Framework for Improving the Quality and Delivery of Psychosocial Interventions • **Recommendation 2-1.** Use the committee's framework for improving patient outcomes through psychosocial interventions to strengthen the evidence base.
Characterize the types of scientific evidence and processes needed to establish the effectiveness of psychosocial interventions. Define levels of scientific evidence based on their rigor.	Chapter 4: Standards for Reviewing the Evidence • Who Should Review the Evidence? • What Process and Criteria Should Be Used to Review Evidence? • Grading the Evidence • Data Sources When Evidence Is Insufficient • How Can Technology Be Leveraged? • **Recommendation 4-1.** Expand and enhance processes for coordinating and conducting systematic reviews of psychosocial interventions and their elements. • **Recommendation 4-2.** Develop a process for compiling and disseminating the results of systematic reviews along with guidelines and dissemination tools.
Define the types of studies needed to develop performance measures for monitoring quality of psychosocial therapies and their effectiveness.	Chapter 5: Quality Measurement • Definition of a Good Quality Measure • Measure Development and Endorsement • A Framework for the Development of Quality Measures for Treatment of Mental Health and Substance Use Disorders • **Recommendation 5-1.** Conduct research to contribute to the development, validation, and application of quality measures. • **Recommendation 5-2.** Develop and continuously update a portfolio of measures with which to assess the structure, process, and outcomes of care. • **Recommendation 5-3.** Support the use of health information technology for quality measurement and improvement of psychosocial interventions. *continued*

TABLE 1-2 Continued

Element of the Statement of Task	Chapters
Define the evidence needed to determine active treatment elements as well as their dose and duration.	Chapter 3: The Elements of Therapeutic Change • An Elements Approach to Evidence-Based Psychosocial Interventions • Advantages of an Elements Approach • Disadvantages of an Elements Approach • **Recommendation 3-1.** Conduct research to identify and validate elements of psychosocial interventions.
Using the best available evidence, identify the elements of psychosocial treatments that are most likely to improve a patient's mental health and can be tracked using quality measures.	Chapter 3: The Elements of Therapeutic Change • An Elements Approach to Evidence-Based Psychosocial Interventions
In addition, identify features of health care delivery systems involving psychosocial therapies that are most indicative of high-quality care that can be practically tracked as part of a system of quality measures.	Chapter 6: Quality Improvement • Consumers • Providers • Clinical Settings/Provider Organizations • Purchasers and Plans • Regulators of Training and Education • Multilevel Quality Improvement and Implementation • **Recommendation 6-1.** Adopt a system for quality improvement. • **Recommendation 6-2.** Support quality improvement at multiple levels using multiple levers.
The following approaches to performance measurement should be considered: • Measures to determine if providers implement treatment in a manner that is consistent with evidence-based standards; • Measures that encourage continuity of treatment; • Measures that assess whether providers have the structures and processes in place to support effective psychotherapy; • Consumer-reported experiences of evidence-based psychosocial care; and • Consumer-reported outcomes using a measurement-based care approach.	Chapter 4: Standards for Reviewing the Evidence • **Recommendation 4-3.** Conduct research to expand the evidence base for the effectiveness of psychosocial interventions. Chapter 5: Quality Measurement • Definition of a Good Quality Measure • A Framework for the Development of Quality Measures for Psychosocial Interventions Chapter 6: Quality Improvement • **Recommendation 6-3.** Conduct research to design and evaluate strategies that can influence the quality of psychosocial interventions.

REFERENCES

AHRQ (Agency for Healthcare Research and Quality). 2011. *Report to Congress: National strategy for quality improvement in health care.* http://www.ahrq.gov/workingforquality/nqs/nqs2011annlrpt.pdf (accessed May 27, 2015).

APA (American Psychological Association). 2015. *Standards of accreditation for health service psychology.* http://www.apa.org/ed/accreditation/about/policies/standards-of-accreditation.pdf (accessed June 18, 2015).

Barth, J., T. Munder, H. Gerger, E. Nuesch, S. Trelle, H. Znoj, P. Juni, and P. Cuijpers. 2013. Comparative efficacy of seven psychotherapeutic interventions for patients with depression: A network meta-analysis. *PLoS Medicine* 10(5):e1001454.

Bauer, M. S. 2002. A review of quantitative studies of adherence to mental health clinical practice guidelines. *Harvard Review of Psychiatry* 10(3):138-153.

Beck, A., A. Rush, B. Shaw, and G. Emery. 1979. *Cognitive therapy of depression.* New York: Guilford Press.

BJS (Bureau of Justice Statistics). 2006. *Mental health problems of prison and jail inmates.* http://www.bjs.gov/content/pub/pdf/mhppji.pdf (accessed March 17, 2014).

Bush, D. E., R. C. Ziegelstein, U. V. Patel, B. D. Thombs, D. E. Ford, J. A. Fauerbach, U. D. McCann, K. J. Stewart, K. K. Tsilidis, and A. L. Patel. 2005. *Post-myocardial infarction depression: Summary.* AHRQ publication number 05-E018-1. Evidence reports/technology assessment number 123. Rockville, MD: AHRQ.

Cherry, D. K., D. A. Woodwell, and E. A. Rechtsteiner. 2007. *National Ambulatory Medical Care Survey: 2005 summary.* Hyattsville, MD: National Center for Health Statistics.

CMS (Centers for Medicare & Medicaid Services). 2014. *CMS measures inventory.* http://www.cms.gov/Medicare/Quality-Initiatives-Patient-Assessment-Instruments/QualityMeasures/CMS-Measures-Inventory.html (accessed May 20, 2014).

Colton, C. W., and R. W. Manderscheid. 2006. Congruencies in increased mortality rates, years of potential life lost, and causes of death among public mental health clients in eight states. *Preventing Chronic Disease* 3(2):A42.

CSWE (Council on Social Work Education). 2008. *Educational policy and education standards.* http://www.cswe.org/File.aspx?id=13780 (accessed June 18, 2015).

Cuijpers, P., F. Smit, E. Bohlmeijer, S. D. Hollon, and G. Andersson. 2010a. Efficacy of cognitive-behavioural therapy and other psychological treatments for adult depression: Meta-analytic study of publication bias. *The British Journal of Psychiatry* 196(3):173-178.

Cuijpers, P., A. van Straten, J. Schuurmans, P. van Oppen, S. D. Hollon, and G. Andersson. 2010b. Psychotherapy for chronic major depression and dysthymia: A meta-analysis. *Clinical Psychological Review* 30(1):51-62.

Cuijpers, P., A. S. Geraedts, P. van Oppen, G. Andersson, J. C. Markowitz, and A. van Straten. 2011. Interpersonal psychotherapy for depression: A meta-analysis. *American Journal of Psychiatry* 168(6):581-592.

Cuijpers, P., M. Sijbrandij, S. L. Koole, G. Andersson, A. T. Beekman, and C. F. Reynolds. 2013. The efficacy of psychotherapy and pharmacotherapy in treating depressive and anxiety disorders: A meta-analysis of direct comparisons. *World Psychiatry* 12(2):137-148.

Drake, R. E., and K. T. Mueser. 2000. Psychosocial approaches to dual diagnosis. *Schizophrenia Bulletin* 26(1):105-118.

Garfield, R. L., S. H. Zuvekas, J. R. Lave, and J. M. Donohue. 2011. The impact of national health care reform on adults with severe mental disorders. *American Journal of Psychiatry* 168(5):486-494.

Grant, S. 2014. *Development of a CONSORT extension for social and psychological interventions.* DPhil. University of Oxford, U.K. http://ora.ox.ac.uk/objects/uuid:c1bd46df-eb3f-4dc6-9cc1-38c26a5661a9 (accessed August 4, 2015).

Grenard, J. L., B. A. Munjas, J. L. Adams, M. Suttorp, M. Maglione, E. A. McGlynn, and W. F. Gellad. 2011. Depression and medication adherence in the treatment of chronic diseases in the United States: A meta-analysis. *Journal of General Internal Medicine* 26(10):1175-1182.

HHS (U.S. Department of Health and Human Services). 1999. *Mental health: A report of the Surgeon General.* Rockville, MD: HHS, Substance Abuse and Mental Health Services Administration, Center for Mental Health Services, National Institutes of Health, National Institute of Mental Health.

_____. 2013. Final rules under the Paul Wellstone and Pete Domenici Mental Health Parity and Addiction Equity Act of 2008. *Federal Register* 78(219):68240-68296. http://www.gpo.gov/fdsys/pkg/FR-2013-11-13/pdf/2013-27086.pdf (accessed May 27, 2015).

Higgins, S. T., and K. Silverman. 2008. Contingency management. In *Textbook of substance abuse treatment*, 4th ed., edited by M. Galanter and H. D. Kleber. Arlington, VA: The American Psychiatric Press. Pp. 387-399.

IOM (Institute of Medicine). 1990. *Medicare: A strategy for quality assurance*, Vol. I. Washington, DC: National Academy Press.

_____. 1999. *To err is human: Building a safer health system.* Washington DC: National Academy Press.

_____. 2001. *Crossing the quality chasm: A new health system for the 21st century.* Washington, DC: National Academy Press.

_____. 2006. *Improving the quality of care for mental and substance use conditions.* Washington, DC: The National Academies Press.

_____. 2010. *Provision of mental health counseling services under TRICARE.* Washington, DC: The National Academies Press.

_____. 2011. *Finding what works in health care: Standards for systematic reviews.* Washington, DC: The National Academies Press.

_____. 2014. *Capturing social and behavioral domains and measures in electronic health records: Phase 2.* Washington, DC: The National Academies Press.

Isett, K. R., M. A. Burnam, B. Coleman-Beattie, P. S. Hyde, J. P. Morrissey, J. Magnabosco, C. A. Rapp, V. Ganju, and H. H. Goldman. 2007. The state policy context of implementation issues for evidence-based practices in mental health. *Psychiatric Services* 58(7):914.

Karlin, B. E., and G. Cross. 2014. From the laboratory to the therapy room: National dissemination and implementation of evidence-based psychotherapies in the U.S. Department of Veterans Affairs health care system. *American Psychologist* 69(1):19-33.

Katon, W., M. Y. Fan, J. Unutzer, J. Taylor, H. Pincus, and M. Schoenbaum. 2008. Depression and diabetes: A potentially lethal combination. *Journal of General Internal Medicine* 23(10):1571-1575.

Kessler, R. C. 2012. The costs of depression. *Psychiatric Clinics of North America* 35(1):1-14.

Kraemer, H. C., G. T. Wilson, C. G. Fairburn, and W. S. Agras. 2002. Mediators and moderators of treatment effects in randomized clinical trials. *Archives of General Psychiatry* 59(10):877-883.

Lin, E. H., W. Katon, M. Von Korff, C. Rutter, G. E. Simon, M. Oliver, P. Ciechanowski, E. J., Ludman, T. Bush, and B. Young. 2004. Relationship of depression and diabetes self-care, medication adherence, and preventive care. *Diabetes Care* 27(9):2154-2160.

Marcus, S. C., and M. Olfson. 2010. National trends in the treatment for depression from 1998 to 2007. *Archives of General Psychiatry* 67(12):1265-1273.

Mark, T. L., K. R. Levit, R. Vandivort-Warren, J. A. Buck, and R. M. Coffey. 2011. Changes in U.S. spending on mental health and substance abuse treatment, 1986-2005, and implications for policy. *Health Affairs (Millwood)* 30(2):284-292.

McGlynn, E. A., S. M. Asch, J. Adams, J. Keesey, J. Hicks, A. DeCristofaro, and E. A. Kerr. 2003. The quality of health care delivered to adults in the United States. *New England Journal of Medicine* 348(26):2635-2645.

McHugh, R. K., S. W. Whitton, A. D. Peckham, J. A. Welge, and M. W. Otto. 2013. Patient preference for psychological vs. pharmacologic treatment of psychiatric disorders: A meta-analytic review. *Journal of Clinical Psychiatry* 74(6):595-602.

Mitchell, A. J., A. Vaze, and S. Rao. 2009. Clinical diagnosis of depression in primary care: A meta-analysis. *Lancet* 374(9690):609-619.

Montgomery, P., S. Grant, S. Hopewell, G. Macdonald, D. Moher, S. Michie, and E. Mayo-Wilson. 2013. Protocol for CONSORT-SPI: An extension for social and psychological interventions. *Implementation Science* 8(99):1-7.

Nakash, O., I. Levav, S. Aguilar-Gaxiola, J. Alonso, L. H. Andrade, M. C. Angermeyer, R. Bruffaerts, J. M. Caldas-de-Almeida, S. Florescu, G. de Girolamo, O. Gureje, Y. He, C. Hu, P. de Jonge, E. G. Karam, V. Kovess-Masfety, M. E. Medina-Mora, J. Moskalewicz, S. Murphy, Y. Nakamura, M. Piazza, J. Posada-Villa, D. J. Stein, N. I. Taib, Z. Zarkov, R. C. Kessler, and K. M. Scott. 2014. Comorbidity of common mental disorders with cancer and their treatment gap: Findings from the world mental health surveys. *Psychooncology* 23(1):40-51.

Peters, R. H., P. E. Greenbaum, J. F. Edens, C. R. Carter, and M. M. Ortiz. 1998. Prevalence of DSM-IV substance abuse and dependence disorders among prison inmates. *American Journal of Drug and Alcohol Abuse* 24(4):573-587.

SAMHSA (Substance Abuse and Mental Health Services Administration). 2012a. *Working definition of recovery.* http://store.samhsa.gov/shin/content/PEP12-RECDEF/PEP12-RECDEF.pdf (accessed September 17, 2014).

_____. 2012b. *State estimates of substance use and mental disorders from the 2009-2010 National Surveys on Drug Use and Health.* NSDUH series H-43, HHS publication number (SMA) 12-4673. Rockville, MD: SAMHSA.

Stein, L. I., and M. A. Test. 1980. Alternative to mental hospital treatment. I. Conceptual model, treatment program, and clinical evaluation. *Archives of General Psychiatry* 37(4):392-397.

Stitzer, M., and N. Petry. 2006. Contingency management for treatment of substance abuse. *Annual Reviews of Clinical Psychology* 2:411-434.

Sudak, D. M., and D. A. Goldberg. 2012. Trends in psychotherapy training: A national survey of psychiatry residency training. *Academic Psychiatry* 36(5):369-373.

Teplin, L. A., K. M. Abram, G. M. McClelland, M. K. Dulcan, and A. A. Mericle. 2002. Psychiatric disorders in youth in juvenile detention. *Archives of General Psychiatry* 59(12):1133-1143.

Thomson, W. 2011. Lifting the shroud on depression and premature mortality: A 49-year follow-up study. *Journal of Affective Disorders* 130(1-2):60-65.

Wang, P. S., M. Lane, M. Olfson, H. A. Pincus, K. B. Wells, and R. C. Kessler. 2005. Twelve-month use of mental health services in the United States: Results from the National Comorbidity Survey Replication. *Archives of General Psychiatry* 62(6):629-640.

Weissman, M. M., H. Verdeli, M. J. Gameroff, S. E. Bledsoe, K. Betts, L. Mufson, H. Fitterling, and P. Wickramaratne. 2006. National survey of psychotherapy training in psychiatry, psychology, and social work. *Archives of General Psychiatry* 63(8):925-934.

Whiteford, H. A., L. Degenhardt, J. Rehm, A. J. Baxter, A. J. Ferrari, H. E. Erskine, F. J. Charlson, R. E. Norman, A. D. Flaxman, N. Johns, R. Burstein, C. J. Murray, and T. Vos. 2013. Global burden of disease attributable to mental and substance use disorders: Findings from the Global Burden of Disease Study 2010. *Lancet* 382(9904):1575-1586. Reprinted with permission from Elsevier.

Wood, E., J. H. Samet, and N. D. Volkow. 2013. Physician education in addiction medicine. *Journal of the American Medical Association* 310(16):1673-1674.

Young, A. S., R. Klap, C. D. Sherbourne, and K. B. Wells. 2001. The quality of care for depressive and anxiety disorders in the United States. *Archives of General Psychiatry* 58(1):55-61.

2

Closing the Quality Chasm: A Proposed Framework for Improving the Quality and Delivery of Psychosocial Interventions

To address its charge, the committee developed a framework for the development of standards for psychosocial interventions that can improve the quality and delivery of those interventions. Figure 2-1 depicts this framework. Adapted from Pincus (2010), the committee's framework identifies the key steps in successfully bringing an evidence-based psychosocial intervention into clinical practice: it highlights the need to support research on the efficacy and effectiveness of interventions, the need to understand the key elements that drive the interventions' effects (Chapter 3), the need to develop a systematic and uniform method for appraising the evidence for the effectiveness of interventions (Chapter 4), the need to develop methods for measuring the quality and outcomes of interventions (Chapter 5), and the need to establish methods for successfully implementing and sustaining these interventions in regular practice (Chapter 6). Central to the framework is the consumer perspective in informing this process.

The framework cycle begins with strengthening the evidence base in order to identify effective psychosocial interventions and their elements. As described in Chapter 1, many evidence-based psychosocial interventions currently exist. While it was beyond the scope of this study to provide a comprehensive review of these interventions, they include a number of psychotherapies, including (but not limited to) interpersonal psychotherapy, dialectal behavioral therapy, cognitive processing therapy, eye movement desensitization and reprocessing, psychodynamic therapy, behavioral couples therapy, problem solving therapy, cognitive-behavioral therapy, social skills training, family-focused therapy, behavioral activation, relaxation training, parent skills training, and motivational interviewing. Evidence-

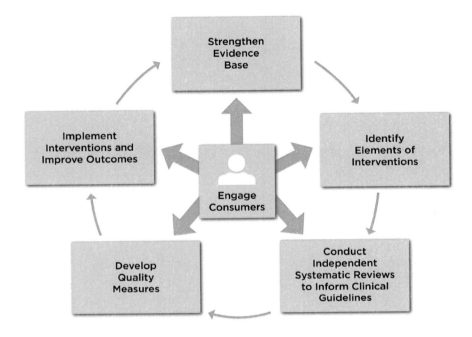

FIGURE 2-1 Framework for developing standards for psychosocial interventions.

based interventions also include behavioral interventions such as contingency management, community reinforcement approach, and exposure and response prevention. The list includes as well ecological interventions such as assertive community treatment, peer-operated support services, peer recovery support services, wellness planning, supported employment, and housing first (IOM, 2010; WHO, 2010).

STRENGTHEN THE EVIDENCE BASE

The data on these interventions are compelling. A number of meta-analyses have established the effects of psychosocial interventions on mental health and substance abuse problems. Psychotherapies in particular have been subject to numerous meta-analyses. In a recent meta-analysis of psychotherapy, the mean effect size across a broad array of mental disorders in 852 trials (137,000 participants) was slightly higher than the corresponding effect size for pharmacotherapies (mean effect size = 0.58 [95 percent confidence interval (CI) = 0.4-0.76] versus 0.40 [95 percent CI =

0.28-0.52]) (Huhn et al., 2014).[1] The effect sizes for psychotherapies varied across mental disorders. The largest effect sizes were for bulimia nervosa (SMD[2] = 1.61, CI[3] = 0.96-2.29), obsessive compulsive disorder (SMD = 1.37, CI = 0.64-2.24), trichotillomania (SMD = 1.14, CI = 0.38-1.89), anorexia nervosa (SMD = 0.99, CI = 0.38-1.6), and binge eating disorder (SMD = 0.86, CI = 0.42-1.3). The effect sizes were still moderate or greater (SMD >0.5) for major depressive disorder, generalized anxiety disorder, social anxiety disorder, posttraumatic stress disorder, and insomnia. The lowest effect sizes were for schizophrenia with psychodynamic therapy (SMD = -0.25, CI = -0.59-0.11) and alcohol use disorders (SMD = 0.17, CI = 0.08-0.26) (Huhn et al., 2014). These effect sizes are based on a variety of different psychotherapies from different theoretical orientations. Several other meta-analyses have been conducted for specific psychotherapies (e.g., cognitive-behavioral therapy, interpersonal psychotherapy, and problem solving therapy), indicating that some therapies are specifically indicated for particular disorders, while others appear to be effective for many different disorders.

Few meta-analyses exist for other types of psychosocial interventions, such as suicide prevention programs, vocational rehabilitation, and clinical case management. However, these interventions have been subjected to randomized controlled trials (RCTs) and have been shown to have positive effects on the intended intervention target.

Although meta-analyses support the use of psychosocial interventions in the treatment of mental health and substance use problems, other studies are needed to further determine the utility of these interventions in different populations and settings. An argument can be made for emphasizing new study designs that yield immediately actionable results relevant to a variety of stakeholders. Tunis and colleagues (2003) describe the need for "practical clinical trials" that address issues of effectiveness—whether interventions work under real-world conditions—as a second step following efficacy studies under the ideal circumstances of an RCT. Pragmatic or practical trials focus on engaging stakeholders in all study phases to address questions related to intervention effectiveness, implementation strategies, and the degree to which an intervention can be conducted to fidelity in a variety of service settings. These studies also address the resources required

---

[1] The effect size is the difference between treatment and control groups and is expressed in standard deviation units. An effect size of 1 indicates that the average treated patient is 1 standard deviation healthier than the average untreated patient. An effect size of 0.8 is considered a large effect, an effect size of 0.5 is considered a moderate effect, and an effect size of 0.2 is considered a small effect.

[2] Huhn and colleagues (2014) measured standardized between-group mean differences (SMDs).

[3] Reported data include CIs.

to implement an intervention. At times, pragmatic trials take advantage of data from electronic health records (EHRs) and insurance claims (Krist et al., 2013). Thus, while a number of psychosocial interventions are supported by existing evidence, many questions remain to be answered with regard to their effectiveness across settings: who is best able to deliver them, what their limitations are, and how they are best implemented.

Given the rigor and time involved in conducting a systematic review of the evidence for psychosocial interventions, this task is beyond the purview of the committee. Chapter 4 provides recommendations for how such systematic reviews should be conducted. The committee refers the reader to published reports from organizations that have reviewed evidence in accordance with the IOM (2011a) report *Finding What Works in Health Care: Standards for Systematic Reviews* (e.g., the Agency for Healthcare Research and Quality, the U.S. Department of Veterans Affairs [VA], and the U.K. National Health Service's [NHS's] National Institute of Heath and Care Excellence). While the reviews discussed here focus on treatment recommendations for specific disease and problem areas, they all include psychosocial/behavioral interventions (when appropriate). The VA and NHS, based on these reviews, have implemented large-scale provider trainings in a number of evidence-based psychosocial interventions, and the authoring organizations note that psychosocial interventions are critical options in treating mental health and substance use disorders.

IDENTIFY ELEMENTS OF INTERVENTIONS

The next step after expanding the evidence base for psychosocial interventions is to standardize them and identify the important elements that drive their effects. These elements, as defined briefly in Chapter 1 and at greater length in Chapter 3, may be either nonspecific (common to all effective psychosocial interventions) or specific to a particular theoretical model or psychosocial approach. Most evidence-based psychosocial interventions are standardized, and these standards are detailed in treatment manuals. Indeed, without these manuals, the implementation of standards for psychosocial interventions would be complicated. For example, the National Registry for Evidence-based Programs and Practices (NREPP) of the Substance Abuse and Mental Health Services Administration (SAMHSA) requires that interventions have a manual or set of guidelines, as well as a training program and a means for measuring quality that tracks to the core competencies in the manuals (SAMHSA, 2015).

Treatment manuals operationalize interventions by describing the theory, procedures, techniques, and strategies they entail. The procedures are detailed with scripts and case examples. Manuals were developed initially to facilitate efficacy studies of psychotherapy, to ensure that therapists were carrying out the treatment under study with fidelity, and to ensure consistency among therapists in how the treatment was delivered. However, manuals have become an important aspect of the implementation of interventions. Without a manual, a guideline, or documentation of how an intervention works, the intervention cannot be deployed as it was developed.

Most manuals have been adapted for different age groups, cultures, disorders, and delivery formats. Sometimes the adaptations have been newly tested, but often they have not. The proliferation of manuals has caused some confusion, and as a result, the manuals often are not widely accepted in clinical practice (Addis and Waltz, 2002). Among the reasons for limited acceptance is the view that the manuals are overly prescriptive and too complicated to follow, and most are not accompanied by evidence-based trainings. When providers are properly trained and supported in an intervention, however, manuals can be useful resources.

Standardization of psychosocial interventions provides an opportunity for identifying the potential nonspecific and specific elements of these treatments. As discussed in Chapter 3, a process for specifying elements will be necessary to improve the impact of psychosocial interventions.

CONDUCT INDEPENDENT SYSTEMATIC REVIEWS TO INFORM CLINICAL GUIDELINES

Once standardized evidence-based psychosocial interventions and their elements have been identified, systematic reviews can be conducted to inform clinical practice guidelines through a methodical, transparent process (IOM, 2011b). As discussed in Chapter 4, centralization of systematic reviews to support the development of guidelines has the potential to minimize the current confusion over which interventions are evidence based and under what circumstances they are most effective. Furthermore, existing standards for systematic reviews may need to be modified for psychosocial interventions to include methods for determining the limits of the interventions, who can be trained to deliver them, and what supports are needed to sustain their quality. Given the cost and time involved in conducting these reviews, innovations from the fields of engineering (e.g., natural-language processing) could be used to expedite the review process.

DEVELOP QUALITY MEASURES

Guidelines based on systematic reviews support decision making among providers and consumers and also form the basis for the development of quality measures that can be used to monitor and evaluate the quality of care in real-world clinical practice settings and ultimately the impact of interventions in improving patient outcomes. Currently, there exist measures of provider competencies, often referred to as fidelity measures, for many evidence-based psychosocial interventions. Like treatment manuals, fidelity measures were developed for use in RCTs to ensure that participants enrolled in a study are actually receiving the treatment under study, but also are not receiving elements from different interventions. A good fidelity tool measures not only providers' adherence to an intervention's strategies and processes, but also the degree to which providers conduct the intervention to competence. It is not enough to know the steps in a treatment; it is important as well to know how to adjust the treatment to meet the needs of the individual consumer without completely abandoning the therapeutic elements that drive the intervention's effect.

IMPLEMENT INTERVENTIONS AND IMPROVE OUTCOMES

A comprehensive quality framework must consider the context in which interventions are delivered. This context includes characteristics of the consumer and the qualifications of the provider. A means for training and credentialing providers in evidence-based treatment is critical to support providers in the use of these interventions. The context for the delivery of interventions also includes the clinic or specific setting in which care is rendered, the health system or organization in which the setting is embedded, and the regulatory and financial conditions under which it operates. Stakeholders in each of these areas can manipulate levers that shape the quality of a psychosocial intervention; shortfalls in the context of an intervention and in the manipulation of those levers can render a highly efficacious intervention unhelpful or even harmful.

ENGAGE CONSUMERS IN THE FRAMEWORK CYCLE

An evidence base demonstrates that consumers bring important perspectives on and knowledge of mental health and substance use problems to psychosocial research and intervention development (Beinecke and Delman, 2008; Berwick, 2009; Deegan, 1993). Their active participation in this process can lead to interventions that address outcomes of most importance to them, improving both adherence and effectiveness (Graham et al., 2014). Consumers are active participants when they offer perspectives and take actions that influence the process of developing and assessing interventions (Checkoway, 2011). As it applies to the committee's framework, consumer involvement is important to identify and formulate research questions for systematic review, help develop guideline recommendations, inform the development of quality measures, and monitor the implementation of interventions.

Active consumer participation has been implemented most comprehensively through a community-based participatory action research (PAR) framework. PAR is a process through which professionals and disadvantaged community members work collaboratively to combine knowledge and action for social change, with community members being able to participate in every stage of the project (Israel et al., 2003).

Implicit in consumer engagement is a thorough consideration of the context for psychosocial interventions, including existing diagnoses, comorbidities, risk factors, social determinants of health, and personal values and preferences. The framework for psychosocial interventions is a complex process, and the committee encourages a broad bio-psychosocial perspective that avoids a siloed approach.

ITERATIVE NATURE OF THE FRAMEWORK

As more evidence emerges from research trials as well as from practical trials based on real-world experience, the cycle of the framework begins anew. Each step in the cycle generates additional research questions and can provide additional evidence. The data systems created for monitoring quality and improving care, for example, can be used in identifying new knowledge about the effectiveness of psychosocial interventions and their elements in different settings or for different populations. Thus, the framework is envisioned as a continuous, iterative process, with each step in the cycle expanding the knowledge base for the development of new and improved standards for psychosocial interventions that can improve patient outcomes.

CONCLUSIONS AND RECOMMENDATIONS

The committee drew the following conclusions about the need for a framework:

The mental health and substance use care delivery system needs a framework for applying strategies to improve the evidence base for and increase the uptake of high-quality evidence-based interventions in the delivery of care.

Broad stakeholder involvement is necessary to develop effective interventions that will lead to improved outcomes for individuals with mental health and substance use disorders.

Recommendation 2-1. *Use the committee's framework for improving patient outcomes through psychosocial interventions to strengthen the evidence base.* **The U.S. Department of Health and Human Services**

should adopt the committee's framework to guide efforts to support policy, research, and implementation strategies designed to promote the use of evidence-based psychosocial interventions. Steps in this iterative process should focus on

- strengthening the evidence base for interventions,
- identifying key elements of interventions,
- conducting independent systematic reviews to inform clinical guidelines,
- developing quality measures for interventions, and
- implementing interventions and improving outcomes.

This is a complex process, and the framework is intended to be used to guide a continuous progression. At each step in the process, systematic research and evaluation approaches should be applied to iteratively expand the knowledge base for the development of new and improved standards for psychosocial interventions that will improve patient outcomes.

Recommendation 2-2. *Require consumer engagement.* The U.S. Department of Health and Human Services and other public and private funding agencies should ensure that consumers are active participants in the development of practice guidelines, quality measures, policies, and implementation strategies for, as well as research on, psychosocial interventions for people with mental health and substance use disorders, and provide appropriate incentives to that end. In addition, family members of consumers should be provided with opportunities to participate in such activities.

REFERENCES

Addis, M. E., and J. Waltz. 2002. Implicit and untested assumptions about the role of psychotherapy treatment manuals in evidence-based mental health practice. *Clinical Psychology: Science and Practice* 9(4):421-424.

Beinecke, R., and J. Delman. 2008. Commentary: Client involvement in public administration research and evaluation. *The Innovation Journal: The Public Sector Innovation Journal* 13(1). http://www.innovation.cc/peer-reviewed/beinicke_7_commenta-_client_public_admin.pdf (accessed February 18, 2009).

Berwick, D. M. 2009. What "patient-centered" should mean: Confessions of an extremist. *Health Affairs* 28(4):w555-w565.

Checkoway, B. 2011. What is youth participation? *Children and Youth Services Review* 33(2):340-345.

Deegan, P. E. 1993. Recovering our sense of value after being labeled mentally ill. *Journal of Psychosocial Nursing and Mental Health Services* 31(4):7-11.

Graham, T., D. Rose, J. Murray, M. Ashworth, and A. Tylee. 2014. User-generated quality standards for youth mental health in primary care: A participatory research design using mixed methods. *BMJ Quality & Safety* 10.1136/bmjqs-2014-002842.

Huhn, M., M. Tardy, L. M. Spineli, W. Kissling, H. Forstl, G. Pitschel-Walz, C. Leucht, M. Samara, M. Dold, J. M. Davis, and S. Leucht. 2014. Efficacy of pharmacotherapy and psychotherapy for adult psychiatric disorders: A systematic overview of meta-analyses. *JAMA Psychiatry* 71(6):706-715.

IOM (Institute of Medicine). 2010. *Provision of mental health counseling services under TRICARE.* Washington, DC: The National Academies Press.

_____. 2011a. *Finding what works in health care: Standards for systematic reviews.* Washington, DC: The National Academies Press.

_____. 2011b. *Clinical practice guidelines we can trust.* Washington, DC: The National Academies Press.

Israel, B. A., A. J. Schulz, E. A. Parker, A. B. Becker, A. J. Allen, and J. R. Guzman. 2003. Critical issues in developing and following community-based participatory research principles. In *Community-based participatory research for health,* edited by M. Minkler and N. Wallerstein. San Francisco, CA: Jossey-Bass. Pp. 53-76.

Krist, A. H., D. Shenson, S. H. Woolf, C. Bradley, W. R. Liaw, S. F. Rothemich, A. Slonim, W. Benson, and L. A. Anderson. 2013. Clinical and community delivery systems for preventive care: An integration framework. *American Journal of Preventive Medicine* 45(4):508-516.

Pincus, H. A. 2010. From PORT to policy to patient outcomes: Crossing the quality chasm. *Schizophrenia Bulletin* 36(1):109-111.

SAMHSA (Substance Abuse and Mental Health Services Administration). 2015. *NREPP reviews and submissions.* http://www.nrepp.samhsa.gov/ReviewSubmission.aspx (accessed May 28, 2015).

Tunis, S. R., D. B. Stryer, and C. M. Clancy. 2003. Practical clinical trials: Increasing the value of clinical research for decision making in clinical and health policy. *Journal of the American Medical Association* 290(12):1624-1632.

WHO (World Health Organization). 2010. *mhGAP intervention guide.* http://www.paho.org/mhgap/en (accessed January 6, 2015).

3

The Elements of Therapeutic Change

This chapter addresses the elements—therapeutic activities, techniques, or strategies—that make up psychosocial interventions. Most if not all evidence-based, manualized psychosocial interventions are packages of multiple elements (see Figure 3-1). As noted in Chapter 1, nonspecific elements (sometimes referred to as "common factors") represent the basic ingredients common to most if not all psychosocial interventions, whereas specific elements are tied to a particular theoretical model of change. Development of a common terminology to describe the elements could facilitate research efforts to understand their optimal dosing and sequencing, what aspects of psychosocial interventions work best for whom (i.e., personalized medicine), and how psychosocial interventions effect change (i.e., mechanism of action). This research could iteratively inform training in and the implementation of evidence-based psychosocial interventions.

AN ELEMENTS APPROACH TO EVIDENCE-BASED PSYCHOSOCIAL INTERVENTIONS

Specific and Nonspecific Elements

Some debate exists as to the relative importance of specific and nonspecific elements. A common factors model for psychosocial interventions suggests that nonspecific elements are the most critical to outcomes (Laska et al., 2014), while other models posit that specific elements are critical above and beyond nonspecific elements (that the specific elements explain a unique portion of the variance in the outcomes) (e.g., Ehlers et al., 2010).

The elements that make up evidence-based psychosocial interventions are clearly specified in measures of fidelity, which are used to ascertain whether a given intervention is implemented as intended in research studies and to ensure that practitioners are demonstrating competency in an intervention in both training and practice. Rarely is a psychosocial intervention deemed sufficiently evidence based without a process for measuring the integrity with which the intervention is implemented. Using a Delphi technique, for example, Roth and Pilling (2008) developed a list of elements for cognitive-behavioral therapy for adult anxiety and depression, which was then used for training and testing of fidelity for the U.K. Improving Access to Psychological Therapies program (Clark, 2011). These elements are shown in Box 3-1.

BOX 3-1
Nonspecific and Specific Elements of Cognitive-Behavioral Therapy for Adult Anxiety and Depression

Nonspecific Elements

- Knowledge and understanding of mental health problems
- Knowledge of and ability to operate within professional and ethical guidelines
- Knowledge of a model of therapy and the ability to understand and employ the model in practice
- Ability to engage client
- Ability to foster and maintain a good therapeutic alliance
- Ability to grasp the client's perspective and world view
- Ability to deal with emotional content of sessions
- Ability to manage endings
- Ability to undertake generic assessment
- Ability to make use of supervision

Specific Elements

- Exposure techniques
- Applied relaxation and applied tension
- Activity monitoring and scheduling
- Using thought records
- Identifying and working with safety behaviors
- Detecting and reality testing automatic thoughts
- Eliciting key cognitions
- Identifying core beliefs
- Employing imagery techniques
- Planning and conducting behavioral experiments

SOURCE: Roth and Pilling, 2008.

The nonspecific elements in a fidelity measure for interpersonal psychotherapy for adolescent depression (Sburlati et al., 2012) are similar, but of course the specific elements differ from those of cognitive-behavioral therapy and reflect the theoretical underpinnings of interpersonal psychotherapy. They include techniques for linking affect to interpersonal relationships (encouragement, exploration, and expression of affect; mood rating; linking mood to interpersonal problems; clarification of feelings, expectations, and roles in relationships; and managing affect in relationships) and interpersonal skills building (communication analysis, communication skills, decision analysis, and interpersonal problem solving skills).

Evidence-based psychosocial interventions for schizophrenia also can be broken down into their elements (Dixon et al., 2010). For example, assertive community treatment for schizophrenia is composed of structural elements including a medication prescriber, a shared caseload among team members, direct service provision by team members, a high frequency of patient contact, low patient-to-staff ratios, and outreach to patients in the community. Social skills training for schizophrenia includes such elements as behaviorally based instruction, role modeling, rehearsal, corrective feedback, positive reinforcement, and strategies for ensuring adequate practice in applying skills in an individual's day-to-day environment.

Cognitive-behavioral therapy for substance use disorders includes elements of exploring the positive and negative consequences of continued drug use, self-monitoring to recognize cravings early and identify situations that might put one at risk for use, and developing strategies for coping with cravings and avoiding those high-risk situations (e.g., Carroll and Onken, 2005). Another example is family-focused treatment for bipolar disorder, which includes elements of psychoeducation, communication enhancement training, and problem solving (Morris et al., 2007).

Elements have been identified for psychodynamic models of psychosocial intervention that are not limited to a specific disorder or set of symptoms. These include a focus on affect and expression of emotion, exploration of attempts to avoid distressing thoughts and feelings, identification of recurring themes and patterns, discussion of past experience (developmental approach), a focus on interpersonal relations, a focus on the therapy relationship, and exploration of fantasy life (Shedler, 2010). For peer support, specific elements can be identified, such as provision of social support (emotional support, information and advice, practical assistance, help in understanding events), conflict resolution, facilitation of referral to resources, and crisis intervention (along with traditional nonspecific elements) (DCOE, 2011).

Specific Elements That Are Shared

Aside from nonspecific elements that are shared across most if not all psychosocial interventions, some specific elements that derive from particular theoretical models and approaches are shared across multiple psychosocial interventions. This is especially the case for manualized psychosocial interventions that are variants of a single theoretical model or approach (such as the many adaptations of cognitive-behavioral therapy for different disorders or target problems or different sociocultural or demographic characteristics). However, sharing of specific elements also is seen with manuals that represent different theoretical approaches, even though they do not always use the same terminology. For example,

- cognitive-behavioral therapy for social anxiety and interpersonal psychotherapy for depression share the element of "enhanced communication skills";
- acceptance and commitment therapy, dialectical behavior therapy, and mindfulness-based cognitive therapy share the element of "mindfulness training";
- a supported employment approach for severe mental illness and problem solving therapy for depression share the element of "behavioral activation";
- contingency management for substance use disorders and problem solving for depression share the element of "goal setting";
- contingency management for substance use disorders and parent training for oppositional disorders share the element of "reinforcement"; and
- "exploration of attempts to avoid distressing thoughts and feelings" is an element of psychodynamic therapy that overlaps with the element of psychoeducation regarding avoidance of feared stimuli in cognitive-behavioral therapy.

Obviously, the further apart the theoretical orientations, the less likely it is that shared elements function in the same way across two interventions. For example, exploration of attempts to avoid distressing thoughts and feelings within psychodynamic therapy functions to identify unresolved conflicts, whereas exploration of avoidance of unwanted thoughts or images in cognitive-behavioral therapy provides the rationale for exposure therapy to reduce discomfort and improve functioning. The discussion returns to this issue below.

At the same time, some specific elements differentiate among manualized psychosocial interventions or are unique to a given manual. For example, the element of "the dialectic between acceptance and change" is

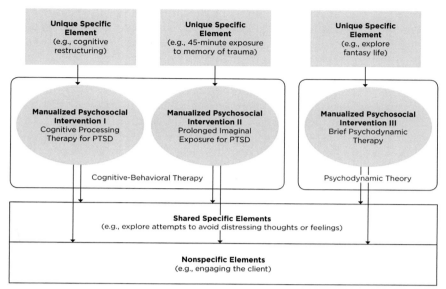

FIGURE 3-1 An example of nonspecific and unique and shared specific elements.
NOTE: PTSD = posttraumatic stress disorder.

generally limited to dialectical behavior therapy, while the focus on "grief, role disputes, transitions, or deficits in order to focus patients on linking their current psychosocial situation with their current symptoms" is largely specific to interpersonal psychotherapy and psychodynamic therapy. Exploration of "fantasy life" is likely to be unique to a psychodynamic approach. Of two interventions that address the needs of the seriously mentally ill, one includes the element of "in vivo delivery of services" (assertive community treatment for the seriously mentally ill [Test, 1992]), and the other does not (illness management and recovery [McGuire et al., 2014]). Figure 3-1 depicts nonspecific elements and specific elements that are shared versus unique for different approaches for the treatment of posttraumatic stress disorder.

Terminology

Recognition of the elements of evidence-based psychosocial interventions highlights the similarities across interventions as well as the true differences. However, this process of discovery is somewhat hampered by the lack of a common language for describing elements across different theoretical models and interventions. Examination of fidelity measures from different theoretical models indicates that different terms are used to describe the same element. For example, "using thought records" in cognitive-behavioral therapy is likely to represent the same element as "mood rating" in interpersonal psychotherapy. Sometimes different terms are used by different research groups working within the same theoretical model; in the packaged treatments for severe mental illness, for example, the notion of "individualized and flexible" is highly similar to what is meant by the term "patient-centered." The field would benefit from a common terminology for identifying and classifying the elements across all evidence-based psychosocial interventions.

ADVANTAGES OF AN ELEMENTS APPROACH

A common terminology for listing elements may offer several advantages for evidence-based psychosocial interventions. A commonly agreed-upon terminology for classifying specific and nonspecific elements would permit researchers to use the same terms so that data could be pooled from different research groups. The result would be a much larger database than can be achieved from independent studies of manualized interventions comprising multiple elements described using different terms. Conceivably, this database could be used to establish optimal sequencing and dosing of elements and to identify for whom a given element, or set of elements, is most effective (i.e., moderation; see below). Elements of medical procedures provide an analogy: many elements are shared across surgical procedures, but surgeries for specific ailments require that the elements be sequenced in particular ways and often in combination with elements unique to an ailment. In addition, it may be possible to connect elements more precisely to purported mechanisms of change than is the case with an entire complex psychosocial intervention. In the future, an elements framework may advance training in and implementation of evidence-based psychosocial interventions. In addition, an elements approach can illuminate both moderators and mediators of the outcomes of interventions (see Figure 3-2).

Moderators

An elements approach for psychosocial interventions may advance the study of moderators of outcome, or what intervention is most effective for a given patient subgroup or individual. The study of moderation is consistent with the National Institute of Mental Health's (NIMH's) Strategic Plan for Research, in which a priority is to "foster personalized interventions and strategies for sequencing, or combining existing and novel interventions which are optimal for specific phases of disease progression (e.g.,

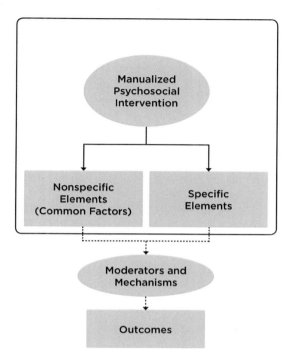

FIGURE 3-2 Moderators and mechanisms of outcomes of psychosocial interventions.

prodromal, initial-onset, chronic), different stages of development (e.g., early childhood, adolescence, adulthood, late life), and other individual characteristics" (NIMH, 2015).

Psychosocial interventions comprising multiple specific elements can be problematic when one is studying moderation, because a complex intervention may include elements that are both more or less effective for a given individual. Thus, for example, an individual may respond differentially to the various elements of an intervention for anxiety disorders (e.g., to "cognitive restructuring" versus "exposure therapy"). Similarly, an individual may respond differentially to "mindfulness training" and "valued actions," which are two elements within acceptance and commitment therapy. At the same time, assessment of moderators of elements (i.e., which element is most effective for a particular patient subgroup) may provide useful information for clinicians and practitioners, enabling them to select from among the array of elements for a given individual. Such investigation could include moderators of elements alone (e.g., for whom exposure to trauma reminders or cognitive reappraisal of trauma is most effective) and of sequences of elements (e.g., for whom cognitive reappraisal is more effective before than following exposure to trauma reminders). Moderator variables might include (1) the disorder or target problem and (2) sociocultural variables such as age, gender, socioeconomic status, and race/ethnicity. It might also be possible to study biomarkers and "aspects of motivation, cognition, and social behavior that predict clinical response" (NIMH, 2015).

Mechanisms

Mechanisms of action could be investigated for each element or sequence of elements across multiple units of analysis (from genes to behavior), consistent with NIMH's Research Domain Criteria Initiative (Insel et al., 2010) and its Strategic Plan for Research, which calls for mechanistic research for psychological treatments. For example, an aim of the Strategic Plan is to "develop objective surrogate measures of outcome and clinical change that extend beyond symptoms, to assess if target mechanisms underlying function, general health, and quality of life have been modified by treatments" (NIMH, 2015). The elements of psychosocial interventions themselves are not mediators or mechanisms. However, elements may have the capacity to be tied more precisely to mechanisms than is the case for a complex psychosocial intervention comprising multiple elements. For example, the element of "cognitive restructuring" relates more closely to the mechanism of attentional bias than does a manual comprising cognitive restructuring, relaxation training, and exposure techniques for anxiety disorders. Similarly, the mechanism of social cognition in schizophrenia may be linked more closely to the element of "social skills training" than to the effects of broader intervention packages such as assertive community treatment or supported employment. Knowledge of mechanisms can be used to hone psychosocial interventions to be optimally effective (Kazdin, 2014). In addition, an elements approach could encourage investigation of the degree to which outcomes are mediated by nonspecific versus specific elements. Although both are critical to intervention success, the debate noted earlier regarding the relative importance of each could be advanced by this approach.

A mechanistic approach is not without constraints. The degree to which mechanisms can be tied to particular elements alone or presented in sequence is limited, especially given the potential lag time between the delivery of an intervention and change in either the mediator or the outcome— although this same limitation applies to complex psychosocial interventions comprising multiple elements. Nonetheless, emerging evidence on the role of neural changes as mechanisms of psychological interventions (e.g., Quide et al., 2012) and rapidly expanding technological advances for recording real-time moment-to-moment changes in behavior (e.g., passive recording of activity levels and voice tone) and physiology (e.g., sleep) hold the potential for much closer monitoring of purported mediators and outcomes that may offer more mechanistic precision than has been available to date.

Intervention Development

The elements approach would not preclude the development of new psychosocial interventions using existing or novel theoretical approaches. However, the approach could have an impact on the development of new interventions in several ways. First, any new intervention could be examined in the context of existing elements that can be applied to new populations or contexts. This process could streamline the development of new interventions and provide a test of how necessary it is to develop entirely novel interventions. Second, for the development of new psychosocial interventions, elements would be embedded in a theoretical model that specifies (1) mechanisms of action for each element (from genes to brain to behavior), recognizing that a given element may exert its impact through more than one mechanism; (2) measures for establishing fidelity; and (3) measures of purported mechanisms and outcomes for each element. Also, new interventions could be classified into their shared and unique elements, providing a way to justify the unique elements theoretically. Finally, the development of fidelity measures could be limited to those unique elements in any new intervention.

Training

When elements are presented together in a single manual, an intervention can be seen as quite complex (at least by inexperienced practitioners). The implementation of complex interventions in many mental health care delivery centers may prove prohibitive, since many such interventions do not get integrated regularly into daily practice (Rogers, 2003). Training in the elements has the potential to be more efficient as practitioners would learn strategies and techniques that can be applied across target problems/ disorders or contexts. This approach could lead to greater uptake compared with a single complex intervention (Rogers, 2003), especially for disciplines with relatively less extensive training in psychosocial interventions. Furthermore, many training programs for evidence-based psychosocial interventions already use an elements framework, although currently these frameworks are tied to specific theoretical models and approaches. For example, the comprehensive program for Improving Access to Psychotherapies (IAPT) in the United Kingdom trains clinicians in the elements of cognitive-behavioral therapy, interpersonal psychotherapy, and brief psychodynamic therapy (NHS, 2008). Conceivably, an elements approach would lead to training in elements of all evidence-based psychosocial interventions, including elements that are shared across these interventions as well as those that are unique to each. In training, each element would (1) be tied to theoretical models with hypothesized mechanisms of action (i.e., a given element may be considered to exert change through more than one purported mechanism); (2) have associated standards for establishing fidelity, which would draw on existing and emerging fidelity measures for evidence-based psychosocial treatment manuals (e.g., Roth and Pilling, 2008; Sburlati et al., 2011, 2012); and (3) be linked with mechanistic and outcome measures.

Implementation

Attempts recently have been made to implement an elements approach for evidence-based psychosocial interventions for children, adolescents, and adults (e.g., Chorpita et al., 2005). One such approach—the Distillation and Matching Model of Implementation (Chorpita et al., 2005) (described in more detail in Chapter 4)—involves an initial step of coding and identifying the elements (i.e., specific activities, techniques, and strategies) that make up evidence-based treatments for childhood mental disorders. For example, evaluation of 615 evidence-based psychosocial treatment manuals for youth yielded 41 elements (Chorpita and Daleiden, 2009). After the elements were identified, they were ranked in terms of how frequently they occurred within evidence-based psychosocial intervention manuals in relation to particular client characteristics (e.g., target problem, age, gender, ethnicity) and treatment characteristics (e.g., setting, format). Focusing on the most frequent elements has the advantage of identifying elements that are the most characteristic of evidence-based psychosocial interventions. Figure 3-3 shows a frequency listing for an array of elements for interventions for anxiety disorders, specific phobia, depression, and disruptive behavior in youth. Figure 3-4 ties the frequency listing for specific phobia to further characteristics of the sample.

In terms of implementation, the matrix of elements (ranked by frequency for different patient characteristics) functioned as a guide for community practitioners, who chose the elements that matched their sample. Whereas Chorpita and colleagues (2005) do not address nonspecific elements (i.e., common factors), an elements approach could encourage practitioners to select nonspecific elements as the foundation of their intervention, and to select specific elements from among those occurring most frequently that have an evidence base for their population (i.e., a personalized approach). With the accrual of evidence, the personalized selection of elements could increasingly be based on research demonstrating which elements, or sequence of elements, are most effective for specific clinical profiles. The

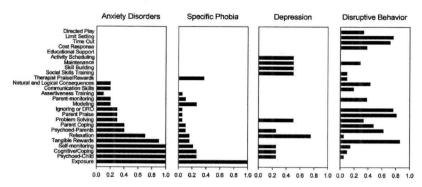

FIGURE 3-3 Intervention element profiles by diagnosis.
NOTE: DRO = differential reinforcement of other behaviors.
SOURCE: Chorpita et al., 2005.

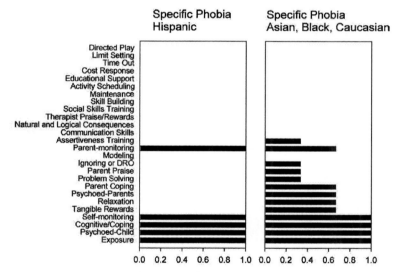

FIGURE 3-4 Intervention element profiles by patient characteristics for the example of specific phobia.
NOTE: DRO = differential reinforcement of other behaviors.
SOURCE: Chorpita et al., 2005.

Distillation and Matching Model of Implementation has been tested, albeit only in youth samples and only by one investigative team. Hence, the results of its application require independent replication.

In a randomized controlled trial, the elements approach was found to outperform usual care and standard evidence-based psychosocial treatment manuals in both the short term (Weisz et al., 2012) and long term (Chorpita et al., 2013). Also, implementation of an elements approach to training in the Child and Adolescent Mental Health Division of the Hawaii Department of Health resulted in decreased time in treatment and increased rate of improvement (Daleiden et al., 2006). The training in Hawaii was facilitated by a Web-based system that detailed the research literature to help clinicians gather information relevant to their particular needs (i.e., which elements are most frequent in evidence-based treatments for a targeted problem with certain sample characteristics). Because the investigative team derived elements from manualized interventions that are evidence based, and because by far the majority of such interventions for child mental health fall under the rubric of cognitive-behavioral therapy, the elements focused on cognitive-behavioral approaches. However, application of a matrix of elements for all evidence-based psychosocial interventions across all targeted problems/disorders and various sample characteristics (e.g., age, gender, ethnicity/race) is likely to provide a larger array of elements that are not restricted to cognitive-behavioral therapies.

DISADVANTAGES OF AN ELEMENTS APPROACH

The elements approach is more closely aligned with psychological therapies than with other community-based psychosocial interventions. In addition, different levels of abstraction may characterize elements from different theoretical models (e.g., structural elements in assertive community treatment versus content elements in cognitive-behavioral therapy). These distinctions may signal the need for different levels of abstraction in defining and measuring elements across psychosocial interventions. Furthermore, an element does not necessarily equate with an ingredient that is critical or central to the effectiveness of an intervention; determination of which elements are critical depends on testing of the presence or absence of individual elements in rigorous study designs. The result is a large research agenda, given the number of elements for different disorders/problems.

As noted above, the function of a shared specific element (such as exploration of attempts to avoid distressing thoughts and feelings) differs across different theoretical models (such as cognitive-behavioral therapy versus psychodynamic therapy). Thus, an elements approach that distills shared elements across different psychosocial interventions fails to recognize the different theoretical underpinnings of the elements. To address this concern, mechanistic studies could evaluate candidate mediators from different theoretical perspectives.

The existing example of implementation of an elements approach in youth samples relies on frequency counts of elements in evidence-based psychosocial intervention research protocols, and is therefore influenced by the number of studies using a given element. The result can be a "frequency bias" when one is making general statements about the importance of any given element.

Finally, only those psychosocial interventions deemed evidence based would be included in efforts to identify elements. Consequently, some potentially effective interventions for which efficacy has not been demonstrated would be omitted from such efforts. Also, because some psychotherapy traditions have not emphasized the demonstration of efficacy, the full range of potentially effective elements might not be identified.

SUMMARY

The committee recognizes the major gains that have been made to date in demonstrating the efficacy of manualized psychosocial interventions through randomized controlled clinical trials. The committee also recognizes that evidence-based psychosocial interventions comprise therapeutic strategies, activities, and techniques (i.e., elements) that are nonspecific to most if not all interventions, as well as those that are specific to a particular theoretical model and approach to intervention. Furthermore, some elements denoted as specific are actually shared among certain manualized psychosocial interventions, although not always referred to using the same terminology, whereas others are unique. The lack of a common terminology is an impediment to research. The committee suggests the need for research to develop a common terminology that elucidates the elements of evidence-based psychosocial interventions, to evaluate the elements' optimal sequencing and dosing in different populations and for different target problems, and to investigate their mechanisms. This research agenda may have the potential to inform training in and the implementation of an elements approach in the future. However, it should not be carried out to the exclusion of other research agendas that may advance evidence-based psychosocial interventions.

CONCLUSION AND RECOMMENDATION

The committee drew the following conclusion about the efforts to identify the elements of psychosocial interventions:

Additional research is needed to validate strategies to apply elements approaches to understanding psychosocial interventions.

Recommendation 3-1. *Conduct research to identify and validate elements of psychosocial interventions.* Public and private organizations should conduct research aimed at identifying and validating the elements of evidence-based psychosocial interventions across different populations (e.g., disorder/problem area, age, sex, race/ethnicity). The development and implementation of a research agenda is needed for

- developing a common terminology for describing and classifying the elements of evidence-based psychosocial interventions;
- evaluating the sequencing, dosing, moderators, mediators, and mechanisms of action of the elements of evidence-based psychosocial interventions; and
- continually updating the evidence base for elements and their efficacy.

REFERENCES

Carroll, K. M., and L. S. Onken. 2005. Behavioral therapies for drug abuse. *The American Journal of Psychiatry* 168(8):1452-1460.
Chorpita, B. F., and E. L. Daleiden. 2009. Mapping evidence-based treatments for children and adolescents: Application of the distillation and matching model to 615 treatments from 322 randomized trials. *Journal of Consulting and Clinical Psychology* 77(3):566.
Chorpita, B. F., E. L. Daleiden, and J. R. Weisz. 2005. Identifying and selecting the common elements of evidence-based interventions: A distillation and matching model. *Mental Health Services Research* 7(1):5-20.
Chorpita, B. F., J. R. Weisz, E. L. Daleiden, S. K. Schoenwald, L. A. Palinkas, J. Miranda, C. K. Higa-McMillan, B. J. Nakamura, A. A. Austin, and C. F. Borntrager. 2013. Long-term outcomes for the child steps randomized effectiveness trial: A comparison of modular and standard treatment designs with usual care. *Journal of Consulting and Clinical Psychology* 81(6):999. Figures 3-3 and 3-4 reprinted with permission from Springer Science.
Clark, D. M. 2011. Implementing NICE guidelines for the psychological treatment of depression and anxiety disorders: The IAPT experience. *International Review of Psychiatry* 23(4):318-327.
Daleiden, E. L., B. F. Chorpita, C. Donkervoet, A. M. Arensdorf, and M. Brogan. 2006. Getting better at getting them better: Health outcomes and evidence-based practice within a system of care. *Journal of the American Academy of Child and Adolescent Psychiatry* 45(6):749-756.
DCOE (Defense Centers of Excellence). 2011. *Best practices identified for peer support programs: White paper.* http://www.dcoe.mil/content/Navigation/Documents/Best_Practices_Identified_for_Peer_Support_Programs_Jan_2011.pdf (accessed May 29, 2015).
Dixon, L. B., F. Dickerson, A. S. Bellack, M. Bennett, D. Dickinson, R. W. Goldberg, A. Lehman, W. N. Tenhula, C. Calmes, R. M. Pasillas, J. Peer, and J. Kreyenbuhl. 2010. The 2009 schizophrenia PORT psychosocial treatment recommendations and summary statements. *Schizophrenia Bulletin* 36(1):48-70.
Ehlers, A., J. Bisson, D. M. Clark, M. Creamer, S. Pilling, D. Richards, P. P. Schnurr, S. Turner, and W. Yule. 2010. Do all psychological treatments really work the same in posttraumatic stress disorder? *Clinical Psychology Review* 30(2):269-276.
Insel, T., B. Cuthbert, M. Garvey, R. Heinssen, D. S. Pine, K. Quinn, and P. Wang. 2010. Research Domain Criteria (RDoC): Toward a new classification framework for research on mental disorders. *The American Journal of Psychiatry* 167(7):748-751.

Kazdin, A. E. 2014. Evidence-based psychotherapies I: Qualifiers and limitations in what we know. *South African Journal of Psychology* doi: 10.1177/0081246314533750.

Laska, K. M., A. S. Gurman, and B. E. Wampold. 2014. Expanding the lens of evidence-based practice in psychotherapy: A common factors perspective. *Psychotherapy* 51(4):467-481.

McGuire, A. B., M. Kukla, M. Green, D. Gilbride, K. T. Mueser, and M. P. Salyers. 2014. Illness management and recovery: A review of the literature. *Psychiatric Services* 65(2):171-179.

Morris, C. D., D. J. Miklowitz, and J. A. Waxmonsky. 2007. Family-focused treatment for bipolar disorder in adults and youth. *Journal of Clinical Psychology* 63(5):433-335.

NHS (U.K. National Health Service). 2008. *IAPT implementation plan: National guidelines for regional delivery.* http://www.iapt.nhs.uk/silo/files/implementation-plan-national-guidelines-for-regional-delivery.pdf (accessed February 12, 2015).

NIMH (National Institute of Mental Health). 2015. *Strategic plan for research.* http://www.nimh.nih.gov/about/strategic-planning-reports/NIMH_StrategicPlan_Final_149979.pdf (accessed February 12, 2015).

Quide, Y., A. B. Witteveen, W. El-Hage, D. J. Veltman, and M. Olff. 2012. Differences between effects of psychological versus pharmacological treatments on functional and morphological brain alterations in anxiety disorders and major depressive disorder: A systematic review. *Neuroscience & Biobehavioral Reviews* 36(1):626-644.

Rogers, E. M. 2003. *Diffusion of innovations,* 5th ed. New York: Free Press.

Roth, A. D., and S. Pilling. 2008. Using an evidence-based methodology to identify the competences required to deliver effective cognitive and behavioural therapy for depression and anxiety disorders. *Behavioural and Cognitive Psychotherapy* 36(2):129-147.

Sburlati, E. S., C. A. Schniering, H. J. Lyneham, and R. M. Rapee. 2011. A model of therapist competencies for the empirically supported cognitive behavioral treatment of child and adolescent anxiety and depressive disorders. *Clinical Child and Family Psychology Review* 14(1):89-109.

Sburlati, E. S., H. J. Lyneham, L. H. Mufson, and C. A. Schniering. 2012. A model of therapist competencies for the empirically supported interpersonal psychotherapy for adolescent depression. *Clinical Child and Family Psychology Review* 15(2):93-112.

Shedler, J. 2010. The efficacy of psychodynamic psychotherapy. *American Psychologist* 65(2):98.

Test, M. A. 1992. Training in community living. In *Handbook of psychiatric rehabilitation,* edited by R. P. Liberman. New York: MacMillan. Pp. 153-170.

Weisz, J. R., B. F. Chorpita, L. A. Palinkas, S. K. Schoenwald, J. Miranda, S. K. Bearman, E. L. Daleiden, A. M. Ugueto, A. Ho, J. Martin, J. Gray, A. Alleyne, D. A. Langer, M. A. Southam-Gerow, and R. D. Gibbons. 2012. Testing standard and modular designs for psychotherapy treating depression, anxiety, and conduct problems in youth: A randomized effectiveness trial. *Archives of General Psychiatry* 69(3):274-282.

4

Standards for Reviewing the Evidence

Reliance on systematic reviews of the evidence base and the development of clinical practice guidelines and implementation tools form the foundation for high-quality health care. However, there is no national, standardized, and coordinated process in the United States for compiling, conducting, and disseminating systematic reviews, guidelines, and implementation materials for use by providers and by those formulating implementation guidance and guidance for insurance coverage. This chapter describes this problem and poses three fundamental questions:

- Who should be responsible for reviewing the evidence and creating and implementing practice guidelines for psychosocial interventions?
- What process and criteria should be used for reviewing the evidence?
- How can technology be leveraged to ensure that innovations in psychosocial interventions are reviewed in a timely fashion and made rapidly available to the public?

As far back as 1982, London and Klerman (1982) suggested that a regulatory body be formed to conduct high-quality systematic reviews for psychosocial interventions, with the aim of providing stakeholders guidance on which practices are evidence based and which need further evaluation. Their proposed regulatory body was patterned after the U.S. Food and Drug Administration (FDA), which subjects all medications and most medical devices to a formal review process and grants permission for marketing.

It is this approval process that informs decisions on which medications and devices can be included for coverage by health plans and should be used by providers as effective interventions. While the concept of having a single entity oversee and approve the use of psychosocial interventions has practical appeal, it has not gained traction in the field and has not been supported by Congress (Patel et al., 2001).

In an attempt to address this gap, professional organizations (e.g., the American Psychiatric and Psychological Associations), health care organizations (e.g., Group Health, Kaiser Permanente), federal entities (e.g., the Substance Abuse and Mental Health Services Administration's [SAMHSA's] National Registry for Evidence-based Programs and Practices [NREPP]), the U.S. Department of Veterans Affairs [VA], nonfederal entities (e.g., the Cochrane Review), and various researchers have independently reviewed the literature on psychosocial interventions. However, the result has been sets of guidelines that often are at odds with one another.[1] Consequently, clinicians, consumers, providers, educators, and health care organizations seeking information are given little direction as to which reviews are accurate and which guidelines should be employed.

A standardized and coordinated process for conducting systematic reviews and creating practice guidelines and implementation tools has the potential to mitigate confusion in the field. Having such a process is particularly important now given the changes introduced under the Patient Protection and Affordable Care Act of 2010 (ACA) and the Mental Health Parity and Addiction Equity Act of 2008 (MHPAEA). As discussed in Chapter 1, under the ACA, treatments for mental health and substance use disorders are included among the 10 essential services that must be covered by health plans participating in health insurance exchanges. However, the act provides insufficient information about which psychosocial interventions should be covered, leaving decisions about covered care to be made by payers, including Medicare, Medicaid, and individual health plans. Without a standardized evaluation process to identify important questions, as well as potential controversies, and to then generate reliable information as the basis for policy and coverage decisions, the quality of psychosocial care will continue to vary considerably (Barry et al., 2012; Decker et al., 2013; Wen et al., 2013). A standardized and coordinated process for reviewing evidence and creating practice guidelines would be useful for various stakeholders, including

---

[1] Existing, well-conducted reviews of the evidence for psychosocial interventions have produced guidelines published by the Agency for Healthcare Research and Quality (AHRQ) (1996), the U.K. National Institute for Health and Care Excellence (NICE) (2015), and the VA (2015).

- educators who train future clinicians,
- clinicians and clinician subspecialty organizations that guide treatment decisions,
- policy makers who drive legislative decisions,
- governmental entities that oversee licensure and accreditation requirements,
- payers that guide coverage decisions and processes, and
- consumers who wish to be empowered in their treatment choices.

Central to the process of compiling the evidence base for psychosocial interventions is the systematic review process. In 2011, the Institute of Medicine (IOM) offered recommendations for conducting high-quality systematic reviews (IOM, 2011). The guidelines broadly identify evidence-based treatments and approaches in health care but generally are not designed to provide the level of detail needed to inform clinicians in the delivery of treatments to ensure reproducibility and a consistent level of quality outcomes—for example, treatment processes, steps, and procedures, and in some cases the expected timeline for response, "cure," or remission. In addition, these guidelines do not address how to evaluate the practice components of psychosocial interventions, specifically, or how to identify the elements of their efficacy. As a result, the IOM guidelines will need to be modified for psychosocial interventions to ensure that information beyond intervention impact is available.

An important challenge in creating a standardized process for reviewing evidence is the fact that systematic reviews as currently conducted are laborious and costly, and can rarely keep pace with advances in the field. As a result, reviews do not contain the latest evidence, and so cannot be truly reflective of the extant literature. In the United Kingdom, for example, the guidelines of the National Institute for Health and Care Excellence (NICE) are updated only every 10 years because of the number of guidelines that need to be produced and the time needed to update the literature, write recommendations, and produce implementation materials (NICE, 2014). Advances in technology may hold the key to ensuring that reviews and the recommendations developed from them are contemporary.

WHO SHOULD BE RESPONSIBLE FOR REVIEWING THE EVIDENCE?

Over the decades, professional organizations, consumer groups, and scientific groups have produced independent systematic reviews, meta-analyses, and practice guidelines for psychosocial interventions. Although these reviews often are helpful to stakeholders, variability in the review processes used by different groups has resulted in conflicting recommendations even when well-respected organizations have reviewed the same body of evidence. For example, two independent organizations reviewed behavioral treatments for autism spectrum disorders and produced very different recommendations on the use of behavioral interventions for these disorders. The National Standard Project (NSP) reviewed more than 700 studies using a highly detailed rating system—the Scientific Merit Rating Scale—and determined that 11 treatments had sufficient evidence to be considered efficacious (NAC, 2009). During the same time period, however, the Agency for Healthcare Research and Quality (AHRQ) sponsored a systematic review of the same literature and concluded that the evidence was not strong enough to prove the efficacy of any treatments for these disorders (AHRQ, 2011). The reason for these differing recommendations lies in how studies were selected and included in the review: the NSP included single case studies using a special process to rank their validity and quality, while AHRQ eliminated more than 3,406 articles based on its selection criteria, according to which only randomized controlled trials (RCTs) were included, and single case studies with sample sizes of less than 10 were excluded.

Having a standardized, coordinated process for determining which interventions are evidence based for given disorders and conditions could mitigate this problem. Two examples of the benefits of such coordination are NICE in the United Kingdom and the VA's Evidence-Based Synthesis Program (ESP). Both employ a coordinated process for conducting systematic reviews and creating guidelines based on internationally agreed-upon standards, and both have a process for evaluating the impact of guidelines on practice and outcomes.

NICE is a nonfederal public body that is responsible for developing guidance and quality standards (NICE, 2011; Vyawahare et al., 2014). It was established to overcome inconsistencies in the delivery of health care across regional health authorities in the United Kingdom and Wales. NICE works with the National Health Service (NHS) to ensure high-quality health care, and is responsible for conducting systematic reviews, developing guidelines and recommendations, and creating tools for clinicians to assist in the implementation of care that adheres to the guidelines. NICE's recommendations encompass health care technologies, treatment guidelines, and guidance in the implementation of best practices. Its guideline process involves a number of steps, with consumers actively engaged at each step (NICE, 2014). A systematic review is called for when the U.K. Department of Health refers a topic for review. A comment period is held so that consumers and clinicians can register interest in the topic. Once there is ample interest, the National Collaborating Center prepares the scope of work and key questions for the systematic review, which are then made available for consumer input. Next, an independent guideline group is formed, consisting of health care providers, experts, and consumers. Internal reviewers within

NICE conduct the systematic review, and the guideline group creates guidelines based on the review. A draft of the guidelines undergoes at least one public comment period, after which the final guidelines are produced, and implementation materials are made available through NHS.

Preliminary reviews of the impact of the NICE process have indicated that it has resulted in positive outcomes for many health disorders (Payne et al., 2013), and in particular for mental health and behavioral problems (Cairns et al., 2004; Pilling and Price, 2006). Recommendations from this body also have informed the credentialing of providers who deliver psychosocial interventions, ensuring that there is a workforce to provide care in accordance with the guidelines (Clark, 2011). In the psychosocial intervention realm, NICE has identified several interventions as evidence based (e.g., brief dynamic therapy, cognitive-behavioral therapy, interpersonal psychotherapy) for a variety of mental health and substance use problems. One result has been the creation of the Increasing Access to Psychotherapies program, charged with credentialing providers in these practices (see Chapter 6 for a full description of this program and associated outcomes).

The VA follows a similar process in creating evidence-based standards through the ESP (VA, 2015). The ESP is charged with conducting systematic reviews and creating guidelines for nominated health care topics. It is expected to conduct these reviews to the IOM standards and in a timely fashion. The VA's Health Services Research and Development division funds four ESP centers, which have joint Veterans Health Administration (VHA) and university affiliations. Each center director is an expert in the conduct of systematic reviews, and works closely with the AHRQ Evidence-based Practice Centers (EPCs) to conduct high-quality reviews and create guidance and implementation materials for clinicians and the VA managers. The process is overseen by a steering committee whose mission is to ensure that the program is having an impact on the quality of care throughout the VA. Regular reviews of impact are conducted with the aim of continuing to improve the implementation process. A coordinating center monitors and oversees the systematic review process, coordinates the implementation of guidelines, and assists stakeholders in implementation and education.

The ESP model has been highly effective in improving the implementation of psychosocial interventions in the VA system (Karlin and Cross, 2014a,b). To date, several evidence-based psychotherapies have been identified and subsequently implemented in nearly every VA facility throughout the United States (see Chapter 6 for details). Program evaluation has revealed that not only are clinicians satisfied with the training and support they receive (see Chapter 5), but they also demonstrate improved competencies, and patients report greater satisfaction with care (Chard et al., 2012; Karlin et al., 2013a,b; Walser et al., 2013).

Based on the successes of NICE and the VA, it is possible to develop a process for conducting systematic reviews and creating guidelines and implementation materials for psychosocial interventions, as well as a process for evaluating the impact of these tools, by leveraging existing resources. The committee envisions a process that entails the procedures detailed below and, as with NICE, involves input from consumers, professional organizations, and clinicians at every step. The inclusion of consumers in guideline development groups is important, although challenging (Harding et al., 2011). In their review of consumer involvement in NICE's guideline development, Harding and colleagues (2011) recommend a shared decision-making approach to consumer support: consumers may receive support from consumer organizations, and should be provided with "decision support aids" for grading and assessment purposes and given an opportunity to discuss with other stakeholders any of their concerns regarding the content of the proposed guidelines, with clear direction on how to initiate those discussions. This approach can be supported by participatory action research training as discussed in Chapter 2 (Graham et al., 2014; Scharlach et al., 2014).

A potential direction for the United States is for the U.S. Department of Health and Human Services (HHS), in partnership with professional and consumer organizations, to develop a coordinated process for conducting systematic reviews of the evidence for psychosocial interventions and creating guidelines and implementation materials in accordance with the IOM standards for guideline development. Professional and consumer organizations, which are in the best position to inform the review process, could work collaboratively with representation from multiple stakeholders, including consumers, researchers, professional societies and organizations, policy makers, health plans, purchasers, and clinicians. This body would recommend guideline topics, appoint guideline development panels (also including consumers, researchers, policy makers, health plans, purchasers, and clinicians), and develop procedures for evaluating the impact of the guidelines on practice and outcomes. When a topic for review was nominated, a comment period would be held so that consumers and clinicians could register interest in the topic. Once the body had recommended a topic for review and the guideline panel had been formed, the panel would identify the questions to be addressed by the systematic review and create guidelines based on the review. For topics on which systematic reviews and guidelines already exist, a panel would review these guidelines and recommend whether they should be disseminated or require update and/or revision.

AHRQ's EPCs[2] are in a good position to assist with the coordination of systematic reviews based on the questions provided by the guideline panels. EPCs are not governmental organizations but institutions. AHRQ currently awards the EPCs 5-year contracts for systematic reviews of existing research on the effectiveness, comparative effectiveness, and comparative harms of different health care interventions for publically nominated health care topics in accordance with the IOM recommendations for conducting high-quality systematic reviews (IOM, 2011). The topics encompass all areas of medicine, including mental health and substance use disorders. The EPCs would report the results of the systematic reviews of the evidence for psychosocial interventions to the guideline panels, which would then create practice guidelines accordingly.

HHS could work with SAMHSA's NREPP (SAMHSA, 2015), AHRQ's National Guideline Clearinghouse (NGC) (AHRQ, 2014), and professional societies and organizations to make guidelines and implementation tools publicly available. Both the NREPP and the NGC were created to coordinate a searchable database of evidence-based practices accessible to any stakeholder, and professional organizations such as the American Psychological Association produce practice guidelines and training materials for association members. Currently, the NREPP is charged specifically with coordinating best practices for mental health and substance use disorders. This organization has been helpful to many mental health policy makers in identifying best practices. At present, however, the NREPP does not use a systematic review process to identify best practices, and as a result, it sometimes labels interventions as evidence based when the evidence in fact is lacking (Hennessy and Green-Hennessy, 2011). If the systematic reviews were conducted by an entity with expertise in the review process (for instance, an EPC), and another entity were charged with coordinating the focus of and topics for the reviews, the NREPP could concentrate its efforts on dissemination of the practice guidelines and implementation tools resulting from the reviews.

Finally, HHS could establish a process for evaluating the impact of the guidelines resulting from the above process on practice and outcomes. In particular, funding agencies charged with evaluating the quality of care (e.g., AHRQ) and the effectiveness of treatment (e.g., the National Institute of Mental Health [NIMH] and the National Institute on Drug Abuse)

---

[2] Current EPCs include Brown University, Duke University, ECRI Institute–Penn Medicine, Johns Hopkins University, Kaiser Permanente Research Affiliates, Mayo Clinic, Minnesota Evidence-based Practice Center, Pacific Northwest Evidence-based Practice Center–Oregon Health and Science University, RTI International–University of North Carolina, Southern California Evidence-based Practice Center–RAND Corporations, University of Alberta, University of Connecticut, and Vanderbilt University. http://www.ahrq.gov/research/findings/evidence-based-reports/centers/index.html (accessed June 21, 2015).

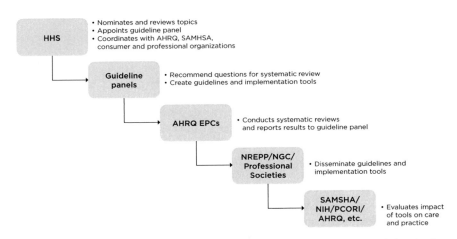

FIGURE 4-1 Proposed process for conducting systematic reviews and developing guidelines and implementation tools.

NOTE: AHRQ = Agency for Healthcare Research and Quality; EPC = Evidence-Based Practice Center; HHS = U.S. Department of Health and Human Services; NGC = National Guideline Clearinghouse; NIH = National Institutes of Health; NREPP = National Registry of Evidence-based Programs and Practices; PCORI = Patient-Centered Outcomes Research Institute; SAMHSA = Substance Abuse and Mental Health Services Administration.

would be poised to fund studies of the impact of the guidelines on practice and outcomes. Ideally, funding would be made available for research and evaluation partnerships among researchers, health care organizations, and consumer groups. The entire proposed process described above is summarized in Figure 4-1.

WHAT PROCESS SHOULD BE USED FOR REVIEWING THE EVIDENCE?

The IOM standards for systematic reviews have been adopted globally, and are now employed in countries with a formal process for determining whether a psychosocial intervention is indicated for a given problem (Qaseem et al., 2012). They also are currently used for guideline development by professional organizations such as the American Psychiatric Association and the American Psychological Association (Hollon et al., 2014). Briefly, the process entails establishing a guideline panel to identify critical questions that guide the systematic review, and ensuring that consumers are represented throughout the process. As noted earlier, the review should be conducted by a group of separate and independent guideline developers.

This group collects information from a variety of sources; grades the quality of that information using two independent raters; and then presents the evidence to the guideline panel, which is responsible for developing recommendations based on the review.

The systematic review process is guided by the questions asked. Typically, reviews focus on determining the best assessment and treatment protocols for a given disorder. Reviews usually are guided by what are called PICOT questions: In (Population U), what is the effect of (Intervention W) compared with (Control X) on (Outcome Y) within (Time Z) (Fineout-Overholt et al., 2005)? Other questions to be addressed derive from the FDA. When the FDA approves a drug or device for marketing, the existing data must provide information on its effective dose range, safety, tolerability/side effects, and effectiveness (showing that the drug/device has an effect on the mechanism underlying the disease being treated and is at least as efficacious as existing treatments) (FDA, 2014).

Although the PICOT and FDA questions are important in determining the effectiveness of psychosocial interventions, they are not sufficient to ensure appropriate adoption of an intervention. Often, questions related to moderators that facilitate or obstruct an intervention's success, such as intervention characteristics, required clinician skill level, systems needed to support intervention fidelity, and essential treatment elements, are not included in systematic reviews, yet their inclusion is necessary to ensure that the intervention and its elements are implemented appropriately by health plans, clinicians, and educators.

It is well known that interventions such as assertive community treatment and psychotherapies such as cognitive-behavioral therapy are complex and may not need to be implemented in their entirety to result in a positive outcome (Lyon et al., 2015; Mancini et al., 2009; Salyers et al., 2003). Beyond the PICOT and FDA regulations, then, important additional questions include the minimal effective dose of an intervention and the essential elements in the treatment package. As discussed in Chapter 3, instead of having to certify clinicians in several evidence-based interventions, a more economical approach may be to identify their elements and determine the effectiveness of those elements in treating target problems for different populations and settings (Chorpita et al., 2005, 2007). The review process also should address the acceptability of an intervention to consumers. For example, cognitive-behavioral therapy for depression is a well-established, evidence-based psychosocial intervention that many health plans already cover; however, it is an intervention with high consumer dropout early in treatment, and early dropout is associated with poorer outcomes (Bados et al., 2007; Schindler et al., 2013; Schnicker et al., 2013).

Reviews also should extract information on the practicalities of implementing psychosocial interventions and their elements. Some psychosocial interventions have been designed for non-mental health professionals (Mynors-Wallis, 1996), while others have been studied across professional groups (Montgomery et al., 2010). Before investing in an intervention, health plans and health care organizations need information about the amount of training and ongoing supervision, basic skills, and environmental supports needed to ensure that clinicians can implement the intervention. Finally, information on the effectiveness of psychosocial interventions across settings is important. As an example, one large study of depression management in primary care found that the intervention resulted in better outcomes when delivered by experts by phone (remotely) than when delivered by local clinicians trained in it (Fortney et al., 2012). Such information helps health care organizations make decisions about the best ways to implement psychosocial interventions effectively.

In sum, systematic reviews for psychosocial interventions should address the following questions:

- **Intervention efficacy**—Is the intervention effective? How is its effectiveness defined and measured? Is the intervention safe? How do its safety and effectiveness compare with those of alternative interventions? What are the minimal effective dose and dose range of treatment (frequency, intensity of setting, and duration)? When should effects reasonably be seen (response to the intervention and remission as a result of the intervention), and when should alternative treatments be considered? What are the essential elements of the intervention?
- **Intervention effectiveness**—Is there evidence that the intervention has positive effects across demographic/socioeconomic/racial/ cultural groups? How acceptable is the intervention to consumers?
- **Implementation needs**—What are the procedural steps involved in the intervention and intervention elements? What qualifications or demonstrated competencies should clinicians, paraprofessionals, or treatment teams have to provide the intervention and its elements effectively? What is the procedure for training the clinician or clinician team? What supports need to be in place to ensure that the intervention and its elements are delivered at a high-quality level and sustained over time? What is the expected number of hours needed in corrective feedback to minimize skill drift? Is supervision required? In what settings can the intervention be deployed? What is the relative cost of the intervention compared with no treatment or alternative treatments?

Grading the Evidence

Asking the right questions for a systematic review is only half the process; identifying the best information with which to answer those questions is just as important. After a guideline panel has determined which questions should be answered by the review, the reviewers must comb the research and grey literature for any information that could be helpful. Once that information has been identified, it is reviewed for its quality with respect to providing definitive answers to the review questions. This review involves grading the quality of the studies' methods and the quality of the evidence generated overall from the existing body of evidence. A number of grading systems for a body of evidence exist, but the one with the most clarity is the Grading of Recommendations Assessment, Development and Evaluation (GRADE) system (Guyatt et al., 2008). The GRADE system ranks the evidence according to the following categories:

- Confidence recommendations: There are several RCTs with consistent results, or one large-scale, multisite clinical trial.
- Future research is likely to have an important impact on the confidence of the recommendations: Only one high-quality study or several studies with limitations exist.
- Further research is very likely to impact the confidence of the recommendations: Only one or more studies with limitations exist.
- Estimate of effect is uncertain: Only expert opinion without direct research evidence is available.

AHRQ adds another important category, called X, when it commissions reviews. This category entails determining whether there is sufficient evidence that the intervention is not harmful.

At issue here is that, as noted earlier, the RCT is considered the gold standard for study designs, and designs that deviate from the RCT are considered less useful in informing recommendations. Yet the RCT method is not appropriate for all questions, such as those concerning implementation and system needs. In some circumstances, moreover, RCTs are not feasible because of pragmatic considerations, such as the lack of a credible control condition or a population's reluctance to engage in randomization, or because of ethical considerations when the only available control is no or poor treatment (Kong et al., 2009; Tol et al., 2008). Suppose the critical question being studied is the number of hours in corrective training needed by a new cognitive-behavioral therapy clinician to maintain fidelity. Unless the aim is to compare needed supervision hours with those for another intervention, the study need not be an RCT, but can be purely observational (Victora et al., 2004). Grading of the extant evidence for a psychosocial intervention, then, should depend on the question being asked, the intervention type, the desired outcome, and the quality to which the methodology of the intervention was employed.

Further, data from field trials and observational studies can complement data from RCTs and mechanistic trials, yet there is little support for this type of research in the arena of psychosocial interventions. While pharmaceutical companies historically have had the resources to field test their interventions, psychosocial interventions often are developed in the field and in academia, rather than by large companies. Whereas agencies such as the National Institutes of Health have served as the primary funders of research evaluating psychosocial interventions, funds for field and observational studies have been constrained by budgetary limitations. More funding is needed to evaluate these interventions so that systematic reviews can be conducted comprehensively.

Data Sources When Evidence Is Insufficient

In the health care domain, there often is incomplete or insufficient evidence with which to determine the effects and processes of interventions. For many psychosocial interventions, compelling evidence supports their effect on symptoms and function in various populations; however, evidence may not be available on relative costs, needed clinician qualifications, or dose of treatment. As discussed above, the evidence for an intervention may be insufficient because funding for research has not been made available. There are three potential solutions when evidence is not readily available to support recommendations on psychosocial interventions: (1) the Distillation and Matching Model (DMM, also called the elements model) (Becker et al., 2015; Chorpita et al., 2007; Lindsey et al., 2014), (2) the Delphi method (Arce et al., 2014), and (3) registries.

The DMM was developed to overcome many problems related to the existence of multiple evidence-based interventions with overlapping elements and the push to have clinicians certified in more than one of these interventions (as described in Chapter 3). The method also was developed to address situations in which a psychosocial intervention is not available for a particular problem. The DMM entails carrying out a series of steps to identify and distill the common elements across existing evidence-based interventions, enabling the identification of best practices for use when no evidence-based treatment is available. The steps in the model are (1) perform a systematic review of all existing interventions, using criteria similar to the IOM recommendations; (2) identify treatment strategies (i.e., elements) within those interventions that are evidence based (e.g., activity scheduling in cognitive-behavioral therapy); (3) identify the elements that are present in at least three existing manuals; and (4) employ intraclass correlations as a means of distilling the remaining, overlapping strategies into final shared elements (Chorpita and Daleiden, 2009). This approach has been applied to child mental health services in California and Hawaii, with positive mental health outcomes in children for as long 2 years posttreatment and with clinicians being able to maintain fidelity to treatment models (Chorpita et al., 2013; Palinkas et al., 2013). The method's major limitation is that it needs additional study. An example of its use is presented in Box 4-1.

The Delphi method—a form of consensus building used traditionally for expert forecasting, such as predicting how the stock market will look based on economic challenges, is a consensus approach to making recommendations about best practices when insufficient evidence is available. The principle behind the method is that forecasts from structured groups of experts are more accurate than those from unstructured groups or from individual predictions. The process includes several steps, beginning with identification of a group of experts who are given, in the present context, questions about what they believe to be evidence-based psychosocial interventions for a particular problem. These experts rarely meet one another during the process. In fact, their identities are kept confidential to minimize the tendency for individuals to defer to those in authority. After a survey group has collected an initial set of responses, it compiles the responses into another survey. That survey is sent back to the experts for further comment, including why they remain out of consensus. The process ends after about four rounds when consensus is reached.

BOX 4-1
Example of the Use of the Distillation and Matching Model
(DMM) for Treating Depression in a 7-Year-Old Boy

Chorpita and colleagues (2007) describe a case in which no evidence-based treatment protocols were available for a 7-year-old boy suffering from depression. Using the DMM approach, they identified interventions for depression for which there was evidence for consumers who matched most of the boy's clinical characteristics. They identified interventions for adolescent depression and from them distilled three elements across manuals—psychoeducation about depression geared toward children, and behavioral activation and relaxation training. They did not include cognitive training because this element, although it often occurred in evidence-based therapies, required intellectual capacity that young children do not possess.

SOURCE: Chorpita et al., 2007.

Registries are another potential source of information when evidence is lacking. Registries are data systems developed for the purpose of collecting health-related information from special populations. Historically, registries have served as sources of information when no RCTs are available, for rare or low-base-rate illnesses (e.g., cystic fibrosis), and for illnesses with no cure (e.g., Alzheimer's disease), and also have been useful in studying the course and treatment response of common illnesses (e.g., diabetes). All consumers with the illness are invited to participate, with no specified inclusion or exclusion criteria. These registries also collect data on any therapies used in any settings. Registries have been employed in evaluating outcomes for the study of issues ranging from the natural history of a disease, to the safety of drugs or devices, to the real-world effectiveness of evidence-based therapies and their modified versions. Box 4-2 outlines the common uses for registries.

Registries are common and widely used in various fields of medicine. As one example, the Cystic Fibrosis Foundation has a registry consisting of health outcomes and clinical characteristics for approximately 26,000 cystic fibrosis patients. This registry has produced important data that now inform treatments used to prolong the survival of these patients. Groups representing other fields of medicine that use registries to inform practice

---

BOX 4-2
Overview of Registry Purposes

- Determining the clinical effectiveness, cost-effectiveness, or comparative effectiveness of a test or treatment, including evaluating the acceptability of drugs, devices, or procedures for reimbursement.
- Measuring or monitoring the safety and harm of specific products and treatments, including comparative evaluation of safety and effectiveness.
- Measuring or improving the quality of care, including conducting programs to measure and/or improve the practice of medicine and/or public health.
- Assessing natural history, including estimating the magnitude of a problem, determining an underlying incidence or prevalence rate, examining trends of disease over time, conducting surveillance, assessing service delivery and identifying groups at high risk, documenting the types of patients served by a health care provider, and describing and estimating survival.

SOURCE: AHRQ, n.d.

are the Society for Thoracic Surgeons, the American College of Cardiology, and the American Society of Anesthesiologists. Both the Health Information Technology for Economic and Clinical Health (HITECH) Act and the ACA support the creation of online registries to improve the quality and reduce the cost of behavioral health interventions, as do health plans, purchasers, hospitals, physician specialty societies, pharmaceutical companies, and patients. As an example, the Patient-Centered Outcomes Research Institute's (PCORI's) PCORnet program[3] has the aim of developing a large and nationally representative registry to conduct comparative effectiveness research.

These approaches to data synthesis when information on psychosocial interventions is not readily available are particularly helpful in identifying directions for future research. When faced with minimal information about the utility of psychosocial interventions in understudied settings and populations, the entity conducting systematic reviews could employ these models to identify candidate best practices and to generate hypotheses about candidate interventions, and could work with research funding agencies (e.g., NIMH, PCORI) to deploy the candidate best practices and study their impact and implementation.

HOW CAN TECHNOLOGY BE LEVERAGED?

The greatest challenge in conducting systematic reviews is the cost and time required to complete the review and guideline development process. A systematic review takes approximately 18 months to conduct, and requires a team of content experts, librarians who are experts in literature identification, reviewers (at least two) who read the literature and extract the information needed to grade the evidence, potentially a biostatistician to review data analysis, and a project leader to write the report (Lang and Teich, 2014). The scope of the review often is constrained by the cost; each question and subsequent recommendation requires its own, separate systematic review. Sometimes new information about treatments is published after the review has been completed, and as a result is not included in the guidelines.

To avoid the cost and timeliness problems inherent in systematic reviews, an entity charged with overseeing the reviews and their products could explore the potential for technology and clinical and research networks and learning environments to expedite the process and the development of updates to recommendations.

In the case of technology, there are many contemporary examples of the use of machine-learning technologies for reliable extraction of information for clinical purposes (D'Avolio et al., 2011; de Bruijn et al., 2011;

---

[3] See http://www.pcornet.org (accessed June 18, 2015).

Li et al., 2013; Patrick et al., 2011; Tang et al., 2013; Xu et al., 2012). Machine learning refers to training computers to detect patterns in data using Bayesian statistical modeling and then to develop decision algorithms based on those patterns. One study has demonstrated that machine-learning technology not only reduces the workload of systematic reviewers but also results in more reliable data extraction than is obtained with manual review (Matwin et al., 2010). Another study employed natural-language processing techniques, preprocessing key terms from study abstracts to create a semantic vector model for prioritizing studies according to relevance to the review. The researchers found that this method reduced the number of publications that reviewers needed to evaluate, significantly reducing the time required to conduct reviews (Jonnalagadda and Petitti, 2013). The application of this technology to ongoing literature surveillance also could result in more timely updates to recommendations. To be clear, the committee is not suggesting that machine learning be used to replace the systematic review process, but rather to augment and streamline the process, as well as potentially lower associated costs.

The use of clinical and research networks and learning environments to collect data on outcomes for new interventions and their elements is another potential way to ensure that information on psychosocial interventions is contemporary. As an example, the Mental Health Research Network (MHRN), an NIMH-funded division of the HMO Research Network and Collaboratory, consists of 13 health system research centers across the United States that are charged with improving mental health care. It comprises research groups, special interest groups, and a large research-driven infrastructure for conducting large-scale clinical trials and field trials (MHRN, n.d.). The MHRN offers a unique opportunity to study innovations in psychosocial interventions, system- and setting-level challenges to implementation, and relative costs. HHS could partner with consortiums such as the MHRN to obtain contemporary information on psychosocial interventions, as well as to suggest areas for research.

CONCLUSION AND RECOMMENDATIONS

Approaches applied in other areas of health care (as recommended in previous IOM reports) can be applied in compiling and synthesizing evidence to guide care for mental health and substance use disorders.

Recommendation 4-1. *Expand and enhance processes for coordinating and conducting systematic reviews of psychosocial interventions and their elements.* The U.S. Department of Health and Human Services, in partnership with professional and consumer organizations, should expand and enhance existing efforts to support a coordinated process for conducting systematic reviews of psychosocial interventions and their elements based on the Institute of Medicine's recommendations for conducting high-quality systematic reviews. Research is needed to expedite the systematic review process through the use of machine learning and natural-language processing technologies to search databases for new developments.

Recommendation 4-2. *Develop a process for compiling and disseminating the results of systematic reviews along with guidelines and dissemination tools.* With input from the process outlined in Recommendation 4-1, the National Registry of Evidence-based Programs and Practices (NREPP) and professional organizations should disseminate guidelines, implementation tools, and methods for evaluating the impact of guidelines on practice and patient outcomes. This process should be informed by the models developed by the National Institute for Health Care and Excellence (NICE) in the United Kingdom and the U.S. Department of Veterans Affairs, and should be faithful to the Institute of Medicine standards for creating guidelines.

Recommendation 4-3. *Conduct research to expand the evidence base for the effectiveness of psychosocial interventions.* The National Institutes of Health should coordinate research investments among federal, state, and private research funders, payers, and purchasers to develop and promote the adoption of evidence-based psychosocial interventions. This research should include

- randomized controlled trials to establish efficacy, complemented by other approaches encompassing field trials, observational studies, comparative effectiveness studies, data from learning environments and registries, and private-sector data;
- trials to establish the effectiveness of interventions and their elements in generalizable practice settings; and
- practice-based research networks that will provide "big data" to continuously inform the improvement and efficiency of interventions.

REFERENCES

AHRQ (Agency for Healthcare Research and Quality). 1996. *Clinical practice guidelines archive.* http://www.ahrq.gov/professionals/clinicians-providers/guidelines-recommendations/archive.html (accessed June 11, 2015).

_____. 2011. *Therapies for children with autism spectrum disorders*. Comparative effectiveness review no. 26. AHRQ publication no. 11-EHC029-EF. http://www.effectivehealthcare. ahrq.gov/ehc/products/106/656/CER26_Autism_Report_04-14-2011.pdf (accessed May 29, 2015).

_____. 2014. *About National Guideline Clearinghouse*. http://www.guideline.gov/about/index. aspx (accessed February 5, 2015).

_____. n.d. *Registries for evaluating patient outcomes: A user's guide*. http://effectivehealthcare. ahrq.gov/index.cfm/search-for-guides-reviews-and-reports/?productid=12&pageaction= displayproduct (accessed June 18, 2015).

Arce, J. M., L. Hernando, A. Ortiz, M. Díaz, M. Polo, M. Lombardo, and A. Robles. 2014. Designing a method to assess and improve the quality of healthcare in Nephrology by means of the Delphi technique. *Nefrologia: Publicacion Oficial de la Sociedad Espanola Nefrologia* 34(2):158-174.

Bados, A., G. Balaguer, and C. Saldana. 2007. The efficacy of cognitive-behavioral therapy and the problem of drop-out. *Journal of Clinical Psychology* 63(6):585-592.

Barry, C. L., J. P. Weiner, K. Lemke, and S. H. Busch. 2012. Risk adjustment in health insurance exchanges for individuals with mental illness. *American Journal of Psychiatry* 169(7):704-709.

Becker, K. D., B. R. Lee, E. L. Daleiden, M. Lindsey, N. E. Brandt, and B. F. Chorpita. 2015. The common elements of engagement in children's mental health services: Which elements for which outcomes? *Journal of Clinical Child and Adolescent Psychology: The Official Journal for the Society of Clinical Child and Adolescent Psychology, American Psychological Association, Division 53* 44(1):30-43.

Cairns, R., J. Evans, and M. Prince. 2004. The impact of NICE guidelines on the diagnosis and treatment of Alzheimer's disease among general medical hospital inpatients. *International Journal of Geriatric Psychiatry* 19(8):800-802.

Chard, K. M., E. G. Ricksecker, E. T. Healy, B. E. Karlin, and P. A. Resick. 2012. Dissemination and experience with cognitive processing therapy. *Journal of Rehabilitation Research and Development* 49(5):667-678.

Chorpita, B. F., and E. L. Daleiden. 2009. Mapping evidence-based treatments for children and adolescents: Application of the distillation and matching model to 615 treatments from 322 randomized trials. *Journal of Consulting and Clinical Psychology* 77(3):566-579.

Chorpita, B. F., E. L. Daleiden, and J. R. Weisz. 2005. Identifying and selecting the common elements of evidence-based interventions: A distillation and matching model. *Mental Health Services Research* 7(1):5-20.

Chorpita, B. F., K. D. Becker, and E. L. Daleiden. 2007. Understanding the common elements of evidence-based practice: Misconceptions and clinical examples. *Journal of the American Academy of Child and Adolescent Psychiatry* 46(5):647-652.

Chorpita, B. F., J. R. Weisz, E. L. Daleiden, S. K. Schoenwald, L. A. Palinkas, J. Miranda, C. K. Higa-McMillan, B. J. Nakamura, A. A. Austin, C. F. Borntrager, A. Ward, K. C. Wells, and R. D. Gibbons. 2013. Long-term outcomes for the Child STEPs randomized effectiveness trial: A comparison of modular and standard treatment designs with usual care. *Journal of Consulting and Clinical Psychology* 81(6):999-1009.

Clark, D. M. 2011. Implementing NICE guidelines for the psychological treatment of depression and anxiety disorders: The IAPT experience. *International Review of Psychiatry* 23(4):318-327.

D'Avolio, L. W., T. M. Nguyen, S. Goryachev, and L. D. Fiore. 2011. Automated concept-level information extraction to reduce the need for custom software and rules development. *Journal of the American Medical Informatics Association* 18(5):607-613.

de Bruijn, B., C. Cherry, S. Kiritchenko, J. Martin, and X. Zhu. 2011. Machine-learned solutions for three stages of clinical information extraction: The state of the art at i2b2 2010. *Journal of the American Medical Informatics Association* 18(5):557-562.

Decker, S. L., D. Kostova, G. M. Kenney, and S. K. Long. 2013. Health status, risk factors, and medical conditions among persons enrolled in Medicaid vs. uninsured low-income adults potentially eligible for Medicaid under the Affordable Care Act. *Journal of the American Medical Association* 309(24):2579-2586.

FDA (U.S. Food and Drug Administration). 2014. *FDA fundamentals.* http://www.fda.gov/AboutFDA/Transparency/Basics/ucm192695.htm (accessed February 5, 2015).

Fineout-Overholt, E., S. Hofstetter, L. Shell, and L. Johnston. 2005. Teaching EBP: Getting to the gold: How to search for the best evidence. *Worldviews on Evidence-Based Nursing* 2(4):207-211.

Fortney, J., M. Enderle, S. McDougall, J. Clothier, J. Otero, L. Altman, and G. Curran. 2012. Implementation outcomes of evidence-based quality improvement for depression in VA community-based outpatient clinics. *Implementation Science: IS* 7:30.

Graham, T., D. Rose, J. Murray, M. Ashworth, and A. Tylee. 2014. User-generated quality standards for youth mental health in primary care: A participatory research design using mixed methods. *BMJ Quality & Safety Online* 1-10.

Guyatt, G. H., A. D. Oxman, G. E. Vist, R. Kunz, Y. Falck-Ytter, and H. J. Schünemann. 2008. Grade: What is "quality of evidence" and why is it important to clinicians? *British Medical Journal* 336(7651):995-998.

Harding, K. J., A. J. Rush, M. Arbuckle, M. H. Trivedi, and H. A. Pincus. 2011. Measurement-based care in psychiatric practice: A policy framework for implementation. *Journal of Clinical Psychiatry* 72(8):1136-1143.

Hennessy, K. D., and S. Green-Hennessy. 2011. A review of mental health interventions in SAMHSA's National Registry of Evidence-based Programs and Practices. *Psychiatric Services* 62(3):303-305.

Hollon, S. D., P. A. Arean, M. G. Craske, K. A. Crawford, D. R. Kivlahan, J. J. Magnavita, T. H. Ollendick, T. L. Sexton, B. Spring, L. F. Bufka, D. I. Galper, and H. Kurtzman. 2014. Development of clinical practice guidelines. *Annual Review of Clinical Psychology* 10:213-241.

IOM (Institute of Medicine). 2011. *Clinical practice guidelines we can trust.* Washington, DC: The National Academies Press.

Jonnalagadda, S., and D. Petitti. 2013. A new iterative method to reduce workload in systematic review process. *International Journal of Computational Biology and Drug Design* 6(1-2):5-17.

Karlin, B. E., and G. Cross. 2014a. Enhancing access, fidelity, and outcomes in the national dissemination of evidence-based psychotherapies. *The American Psychologist* 69(7):709-711.

_____. 2014b. From the laboratory to the therapy room: National dissemination and implementation of evidence-based psychotherapies in the U.S. Department of Veterans Affairs health care system. *The American Psychologist* 69(1):19-33.

Karlin, B. E., R. D. Walser, J. Yesavage, A. Zhang, M. Trockel, and C. B. Taylor. 2013a. Effectiveness of acceptance and commitment therapy for depression: Comparison among older and younger veterans. *Aging & Mental Health* 17(5):555-563.

Karlin, B. E., M. Trockel, C. B. Taylor, J. Gimeno, and R. Manber. 2013b. National dissemination of cognitive-behavioral therapy for insomnia in veterans: Therapist- and patient-level outcomes. *Journal of Consulting and Clinical Psychology* 81(5):912-917.

Kong, E. H., L. K. Evans, and J. P. Guevara. 2009. Nonpharmacological intervention for agitation in dementia: A systematic review and meta-analysis. *Aging & Mental Health* 13(4):512-520.

Lang, L. A., and S. T. Teich. 2014. A critical appraisal of the systematic review process: Systematic reviews of zirconia single crowns. *The Journal of Prosthetic Dentistry* 111(6): 476-484.

Li, Q., H. Zhai, L. Deleger, T. Lingren, M. Kaiser, L. Stoutenborough, and I. Solti. 2013. A sequence labeling approach to link medications and their attributes in clinical notes and clinical trial announcements for information extraction. *Journal of the American Medical Informatics Association* 20(5):915-921.

Lindsey, M. A., N. E. Brandt, K. D. Becker, B. R. Lee, R. P. Barth, E. L. Daleiden, and B. F. Chorpita. 2014. Identifying the common elements of treatment engagement interventions in children's mental health services. *Clinical Child and Family Psychology Review* 17(3):283-298.

London, P., and G. L. Klerman. 1982. Evaluating psychotherapy. *American Journal of Psychiatry* 139(6):709-717.

Lyon, A. R., S. Dorsey, M. Pullmann, J. Silbaugh-Cowdin, and L. Berliner. 2015. Clinician use of standardized assessments following a common elements psychotherapy training and consultation program. *Administration and Policy in Mental Health* 42(1):47-60.

Mancini, A. D., L. L. Moser, R. Whitley, G. J. McHugo, G. R. Bond, M. T. Finnerty, and B. J. Burns. 2009. Assertive community treatment: Facilitators and barriers to implementation in routine mental health settings. *Psychiatric Services* 60(2):189-195.

Matwin, S., A. Kouznetsov, D. Inkpen, O. Frunza, and P. O'Blenis. 2010. A new algorithm for reducing the workload of experts in performing systematic reviews. *Journal of the American Medical Informatics Association* 17(4):446-453.

MHRN (Mental Health Research Network). n.d. *About.* https://sites.google.com/a/mhresearch network.org/mhrn/home/about-us (accessed February 6, 2015).

Montgomery, E. C., M. E. Kunik, N. Wilson, M. A. Stanley, and B. Weiss. 2010. Can paraprofessionals deliver cognitive-behavioral therapy to treat anxiety and depressive symptoms? *Bulletin of the Menninger Clinic* 74(1):45-62.

Mynors-Wallis, L. 1996. Problem-solving treatment: Evidence for effectiveness and feasibility in primary care. *International Journal of Psychiatry in Medicine* 26(3):249-262.

NAC (National Autism Center). 2009. *National standards report: Phase 1.* http://dlr.sd.gov/ autism/documents/nac_standards_report_2009.pdf (accessed February 21, 2015).

NICE (National Institute for Health and Clinical Excellence). 2011. *Common mental health disorders: Identification and pathways to care.* Leicester, UK: British Psychological Society.

_____. 2014. *Developing NICE guidelines: The manual.* https://www.nice.org.uk/article/ pmg20/chapter/1-Introduction-and-overview (accessed February 5, 2014).

_____. 2015. *Guidance list.* http://www.nice.org.uk/guidance/published?type=Guidelines (accessed June 11, 2015).

Palinkas, L. A., J. R. Weisz, B. F. Chorpita, B. Levine, A. F. Garland, K. E. Hoagwood, and J. Landsverk. 2013. Continued use of evidence-based treatments after a randomized controlled effectiveness trial: A qualitative study. *Psychiatric Services* 64(11):1110-1118.

Patel, V. L., J. F. Arocha, M. Diermeier, R. A. Greenes, and E. H. Shortliffe. 2001. Methods of cognitive analysis to support the design and evaluation of biomedical systems: The case of clinical practice guidelines. *Journal of Biomedical Informatics* 34(1):52-66.

Patrick, J. D., D. H. Nguyen, Y. Wang, and M. Li. 2011. A knowledge discovery and reuse pipeline for information extraction in clinical notes. *Journal of the American Medical Informatics Association* 18(5):574-579.

Payne, H., N. Clarke, R. Huddart, C. Parker, J. Troup, and J. Graham. 2013. Nasty or nice? Findings from a U.K. survey to evaluate the impact of the National Institute for Health and Clinical Excellence (NICE) clinical guidelines on the management of prostate cancer. *Clinical Oncology* 25(3):178-189.

Pilling, S., and K. Price. 2006. Developing and implementing clinical guidelines: Lessons from the NICE schizophrenia guideline. *Epidemiologia e Psichiatria Sociale* 15(2):109-116.

Qaseem, A., F. Forland, F. Macbeth, G. Ollenschläger, S. Phillips, and P. van der Wees. 2012. Guidelines international network: Toward international standards for clinical practice guidelines. *Annals of Internal Medicine* 156(7):525-531.

Salyers, M. P., G. R. Bond, G. B. Teague, J. F. Cox, M. E. Smith, M. L. Hicks, and J. I. Koop. 2003. Is it ACT yet? Real-world examples of evaluating the degree of implementation for assertive community treatment. *Journal of Behavioral Health Services & Research* 30(3):304-320.

SAMHSA (Substance Abuse and Mental Health Services Administration). 2015. *About SAMHSA's National Registry of Evidence-based Programs and Practices.* http://www.nrepp.samhsa.gov/AboutNREPP.aspx (accessed February 5, 2015).

Scharlach, A. E., C. L. Graham, and C. Berridge. 2014. An integrated model of co-ordinated community-based care. *Gerontologist* doi:10.1093/geront/gnu075.

Schindler, A., W. Hiller, and M. Witthoft. 2013. What predicts outcome, response, and drop-out in CBT of depressive adults? A naturalistic study. *Behavioural and Cognitive Psychotherapy* 41(3):365-370.

Schnicker, K., W. Hiller, and T. Legenbauer. 2013. Drop-out and treatment outcome of outpatient cognitive-behavioral therapy for anorexia nervosa and bulimia nervosa. *Comprehensive Psychiatry* 54(7):812-823.

Tang, B., Y. Wu, M. Jiang, Y. Chen, J. C. Denny, and H. Xu. 2013. A hybrid system for temporal information extraction from clinical text. *Journal of the American Medical Informatics Association* 20(5):828-835.

Tol, W. A., I. H. Komproe, D. Susanty, M. J. Jordans, R. D. Macy, and J. T. De Jong. 2008. School-based mental health intervention for children affected by political violence in Indonesia: A cluster randomized trial. *Journal of the American Medical Association* 300(6):655-662.

VA (U.S. Department of Veterans Affairs). 2015. *Health Services Research and Development: Evidence-Based Synthesis Program.* http://www.hsrd.research.va.gov/publications/esp (accessed February 5, 2015).

Victora, C. G., J. P. Habicht, and J. Bryce. 2004. Evidence-based public health: Moving beyond randomized trials. *American Journal of Public Health* 94(3):400-405.

Vyawahare, B., N. Hallas, M. Brookes, R. S. Taylor, and S. Eldabe. 2014. Impact of the National Institute for Health and Care Excellence (NICE) guidance on medical technology uptake: Analysis of the uptake of spinal cord stimulation in England 2008-2012. *BMJ Open* 4(1):e004182.

Walser, R. D., B. E. Karlin, M. Trockel, B. Mazina, and C. Barr Taylor. 2013. Training in and implementation of Acceptance and Commitment Therapy for depression in the Veterans Health Administration: Therapist and patient outcomes. *Behaviour Research and Therapy* 51(9):555-563.

Wen, H., J. R. Cummings, J. M. Hockenberry, L. M. Gaydos, and B. G. Druss. 2013. State parity laws and access to treatment for substance use disorder in the United States: Implications for federal parity legislation. *JAMA Psychiatry* 70(12):1355-1362.

Xu, Y., K. Hong, J. Tsujii, and E. I. Chang. 2012. Feature engineering combined with machine learning and rule-based methods for structured information extraction from narrative clinical discharge summaries. *Journal of the American Medical Informatics Association* 19(5):824-832.

5

Quality Measurement

The Patient Protection and Affordable Care Act (ACA) has set the stage for transformation of the health care system. This transformation includes change in what the nation wants from health care as well as in how care is paid for. New care delivery systems and payment reforms require measures for tracking the performance of the health care system. Quality measures are among the critical tools for health care providers and organizations during the process of transformation and improvement (Conway and Clancy, 2009). Quality measures also play a critical role in the implementation and monitoring of innovative interventions and programs. This chapter begins by defining a good quality measure. It then reviews the process for measure development and endorsement and the existing landscape of quality measures for treatment of mental health and substance use (MH/SU) disorders. Next, the chapter details a framework for the development of quality measures—structural, process, and outcome measures—for psychosocial interventions, including the advantages, disadvantages, opportunities, and challenges associated with each. The final section presents the committee's recommendations on quality measurement.

DEFINITION OF A GOOD QUALITY MEASURE

The Institute of Medicine (IOM) defines *quality of care* as "the degree to which health care services for individuals and populations increase the likelihood of desired health outcomes and are consistent with current professional knowledge" (IOM, 1990, p. 21). *Quality measures* are tools for quantifying a component or aspect of health care and comparing it against an evidence-based criterion (NQMC, 2014).

Quality measures are used at multiple levels of the health care system—clinicians, practices, clinics, organizations, and health plans—and for multiple purposes, including clinical care, quality improvement, and accountability. At the patient level, quality measures can address the patient experience of care and issues that are important to the patient's treatment plan. At the care team or clinician level, quality measures can be used to assess the effectiveness and efficiency of care and inform quality improvement efforts. At the organization level (such as a health plan or delivery system), quality measures can address how well the organization supports effective care delivery—for example, by being used to assess the availability of trained staff. At the policy level, quality measures can be used to assess the effect of policies, regulations, or payment methodologies in supporting effective care. And at the level of the clinician or care team and organization, quality measures often are used for accountability purposes—for example, through public reporting to support consumer or purchaser decision making or as the basis for payment or other nonfinancial incentives (such as preferential network status).

Quality measures can address structure, process, and outcomes (Donabedian, 1980). Structure measures assess the capacity of organizations and providers to provide effective/evidence-based care likely to achieve favorable outcomes. Structure measures typically include features related to the presence of policies and procedures, personnel, physical plant, and information technology capacity and functionality. Process measures are used to assess how well a health care service provided to a patient adheres to recommendations for clinical practice based on evidence or consensus. Process measures may also be used to assess accessibility of services. Health outcomes are the "effects of care on the health status of patients and populations," which include the patient's improved health knowledge, health-related behavior, and satisfaction with care in addition to specific relevant health measures (Donabedian, 1988).

MEASURE DEVELOPMENT AND ENDORSEMENT

Various organizations have defined desirable criteria for quality measures. These criteria address such questions as importance (e.g., whether the condition or topic is common or costly and whether it has a large impact on outcomes), the evidence base or rationale supporting the measure, the scientific soundness of the measure (e.g., whether it provides valid and reliable results), the feasibility of and effort required for reporting, and the degree to which the information provided is useful for a variety of stakeholders

---

BOX 5-1
National Quality Forum's Criteria for
Evaluation of Quality Measures

Importance to measure and report—measures address those aspects with the greatest potential for driving improvements; if measures are not important, the other criteria are less meaningful (must-pass)

Scientific acceptability of measure properties—the goal is to enable valid conclusions about quality; if measures are not reliable and valid, there is a risk of misclassification and improper interpretation (must-pass)

Feasibility—ideally, administering the measures should impose as little burden as possible; if administration is not feasible, consider alternative approaches

Usability and use—the goal is to be able to use endorsed measures for decisions related to accountability and improvement

Harmonization and selection of best-in-class—the steward attests that a measure's specifications have been standardized for related measures with the same focus and that issues with competing measures have been considered and addressed

SOURCE: Burstin, 2014.

(McGlynn, 1998; NQF, 2014c; NQMC, 2014). As an example, Box 5-1 lists the criteria for evaluation of quality measures of the National Quality Forum (NQF). To illustrate, some of the most widely used quality measures address care for diabetes, including control of blood sugar and annual testing to detect complications that can lead to blindness, renal failure, and amputations. These measures are considered important because diabetes is a common and costly disease, and because there is strong evidence that maintaining glycemic control can minimize the disease's complications and that early identification of these complications can lessen further deterioration (Vinik and Vinik, 2003). Furthermore, the information needed to report these measures can be captured reliably and validly from existing data in administrative claims, laboratory results, and medical records, thus making the measures feasible and scientifically sound. Multiple stakeholders also can use the measures for targeting quality improvement efforts and for engaging patients in self-care.

The process for developing quality measures includes specific efforts to address each of these criteria. Key steps include evaluating the impact of the quality concern and the evidence for the likely effectiveness of specific

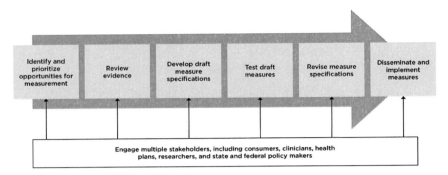

FIGURE 5-1 The development process for quality measures.
SOURCE: Adapted from Byron et al., 2014.

interventions or actions by the health care system to address the concern, specifying in detail how to calculate the measure, and testing the measure (see Figure 5-1) (Byron et al., 2014; CMS, n.d.). Input from multiple stakeholders throughout the process is considered essential (Byron et al., 2014; NQF, 2014a); stakeholders include consumers (whose care is the focus of measurement and who will use quality information to inform their decisions), experts in the topic area of the measures, those who will implement the measures (government, purchasers), and those who will be evaluated by the measures (providers, health plans). Input may be obtained through ongoing advice from a multistakeholder panel, solicitation of input from key stakeholders, or broad input from a public comment period. While consumer involvement as stakeholders in advising on measure concepts has occurred in some settings, consumer participation on measure development teams has been limited.

A large number of quality measures have been developed by accrediting organizations such as the Joint Commission (for hospitals) and the National Committee for Quality Assurance (NCQA, for health plans). Physician groups also have developed measures; examples include the Physician Consortium for Performance Improvement, convened by the American Medical Association, and specialty societies such as the American College of Surgeons and the American Society for Clinical Oncology. Recently, the federal government has assumed a large role in measure development to support implementation of the ACA. Agencies of the U.S. Department of Health and Human Services (HHS) have contracted with a variety of organizations for the development of new measures (e.g., for the Centers for Medicare & Medicaid Services' [CMS's] electronic health records [EHRs] incentive program or for inpatient psychiatric facilities). Additionally, the Children's Health Insurance Program Reauthorization Act (CHIPRA) called for an unprecedented investment in pediatric quality measures, and many measures addressing mental health conditions are in development through that effort (AHRQ, 2010).

Given the growth in quality measurement efforts and the number of quality measures, CMS has worked to coordinate these efforts so as to avoid undue burden or mixed signals and ensure that measures are useful for multiple stakeholders (Frank, 2014; Ling, 2014). Two mechanisms supporting the rationalization of measurement and the reduction of duplication are (1) the use of a multistakeholder consensus-based process for endorsing measures, and (2) prioritization of measures for public programs.

Currently, HHS contracts with NQF, an independent, nonprofit consensus-based entity, to prioritize, endorse, and maintain valid quality performance measures. To implement its endorsement process, NQF issues calls for measures in specific content areas and convenes multistakeholder committees to review candidate measures against the criteria listed earlier in Box 5-1. The committees' recommendations are posted for public comment, and final recommendations are made by NQF's governing committee (NQF, 2014a). Endorsement lasts 3 years, but annual updates are required, and measures can be reevaluated when new, competing measures are proposed.

The second mechanism—prioritization of measures for public programs—is formally incorporated in the ACA. The Measures Application Partnership (MAP), convened by NQF, provides multistakeholder input prior to federal rulemaking on measures to be used in federal public reporting and performance-based payment programs. In particular, the role of the MAP is to align measures used in public and private programs and to prioritize areas for new measure development (NQF, 2014b).

THE EXISTING LANDSCAPE OF QUALITY MEASURES FOR TREATMENT OF MENTAL HEALTH AND SUBSTANCE USE DISORDERS

To date, quality measures are lacking for key areas of MH/SU treatment. Of the 55 nationally endorsed measures related to MH/SU, just 2 address a psychosocial intervention (both dealing with intervention for substance use) (see Table 5-1). An international review of quality measures in mental health similarly showed the lack of measures for psychosocial interventions, with fewer than 10 percent of identified measures being considered applicable to these interventions (Fisher et al., 2013). The small number of nationally endorsed quality measures addressing MH/SU reflects both limitations in the evidence base for what treatments are effective at achieving improvements in patient outcomes and challenges faced in obtaining the detailed information necessary to support quality measurement from

TABLE 5-1 Measures Related to Mental Health and Substance Use Endorsed by the National Quality Forum as of July 2015

Measure Title	NQF#	Type
Depression Response at Six Months—Progress Toward Remission	1884	Outcome
Depression Response at Twelve Months—Progress Toward Remission	1885	Outcome
Depression Remission at Six Months	0711	Outcome
Depression Remission at Twelve Months	0710	Outcome
Inpatient Consumer Survey (ICS) (consumer evaluation of inpatient behavioral health care services)	0726	Outcome
Pediatric Symptom Checklist (PSC)	0722	Outcome
Controlling High Blood Pressure for People with Serious Mental Illness	2602	Outcome
Diabetes Care for People with Serious Mental Illness: Blood Pressure Control (<140/90 mm Hg)	2606	Outcome
Diabetes Care for People with Serious Mental Illness: Hemoglobin A1c (HbA1c) Poor Control (>9.0%)	2607	Outcome
Diabetes Care for People with Serious Mental Illness: Hemoglobin A1c (HbA1c) Control (<8.0%)	2608	Outcome
Promoting Healthy Development Survey (PHDS)	0011	Outcome
Experience of Care and Health Outcomes (ECHO) Survey (behavioral health, managed care versions)	0008	Outcome
Adult Current Smoking Prevalence	2020	Outcome[a]
Depression Utilization of the PHQ-9 Tool	0712	Process
Antidepressant Medication Management (AMM)	0105	Process
Adult Major Depressive Disorder (MDD): Suicide Risk Assessment	0104	Process
Child and Adolescent Major Depressive Disorder: Diagnostic Evaluation	1364	Process
Child and Adolescent Major Depressive Disorder: Suicide Risk Assessment	1365	Process
Developmental Screening in the First Three Years of Life	1448	Process
SUB-1 Alcohol Use Screening	1661	Process
SUB-2 Alcohol Use Brief Intervention Provided or Offered and SUB-2a Alcohol Use Brief Intervention	1663	Process

TABLE 5-1 Continued

Measure Title	NQF#	Type
SUB-3 Alcohol and Other Drug Use Disorder Treatment Provided or Offered at Discharge and SUB-3a Alcohol and Other Drug Use Disorder Treatment at Discharge	1664	Process
Adherence to Antipsychotic Medications for Individuals with Schizophrenia	1879	Process
Adherence to Mood Stabilizers for Individuals with Bipolar I Disorder	1880	Process
Antipsychotic Use in Persons with Dementia	2111	Process
HBIPS-1 Admission Screening	1922	Process
Follow-up After Hospitalization for Schizophrenia (7- and 30-day)	1937	Process
HBIPS-5 Patients Discharged on Multiple Antipsychotic Medications with Appropriate Justification	0560	Process
HBIPS-6 Post-Discharge Continuing Care Plan Created	0557	Process
HBIPS-7 Post-Discharge Continuing Care Plan Transmitted to Next Level of Care Provider Upon Discharge	0558	Process
HBIPS-2 Hours of Physical Restraint Use	0640	Process
HBIPS-3 Hours of Seclusion Use	0641	Process
Cardiovascular Health Screening for People with Schizophrenia or Bipolar Disorder Who Are Prescribed Antipsychotic Medications	1927	Process
Diabetes Screening for People with Schizophrenia or Bipolar Disorder Who Are Using Antipsychotic Medications (SSD)	1932	Process
Cardiovascular Monitoring for People with Cardiovascular Disease and Schizophrenia (SMC)	1933	Process
Diabetes Monitoring for People with Diabetes and Schizophrenia (SMD)	1934	Process
Substance Use Screening and Intervention Composite	2597	Process
Antipsychotic Use in Children Under 5 Years Old	2337	Process
Alcohol Screening and Follow-up for People with Serious Mental Illness	2599	Process
Tobacco Use Screening and Follow-up for People with Serious Mental Illness or Alcohol or Other Drug Dependence	2600	Process
Body Mass Index Screening and Follow-up for People with Serious Mental Illness	2601	Process
Diabetes Care for People with Serious Mental Illness: Hemoglobin A1c (HbA1c) Testing	2603	Process

continued

TABLE 5-1 Continued

Measure Title	NQF#	Type
Diabetes Care for People with Serious Mental Illness: Medical Attention for Nephropathy	2604	Process
Follow-up After Discharge from the Emergency Department for Mental Health or Alcohol or Other Drug Dependence	2605	Process
Diabetes Care for People with Serious Mental Illness: Eye Exam	2609	Process
Initiation and Engagement of Alcohol and Other Drug Dependence Treatment (IET)	0004	Process
Preventive Care and Screening: Unhealthy Alcohol Use: Screening and Brief Counseling	2152	Process
Preventive Care and Screening: Screening for Clinical Depression and Follow-up Plan	0418	Process
Follow-up Care for Children Prescribed ADHD Medication (ADD)	0108	Process
Depression Assessment Conducted	0518	Process
Follow-up After Hospitalization for Mental Illness (FUH)	0576	Process
Developmental Screening Using a Parent Completed Screening Tool (Parent report, Children 0-5)	1385	Process
TOB-1 Tobacco Use Screening	1651	Process
TOB-2 Tobacco Use Treatment Provided or Offered and the Subset Measure TOB-2a Tobacco Use Treatment	1654	Process
TOB-3 Tobacco Use Treatment Provided or Offered at Discharge and the Subset Measure TOB-3a Tobacco Use Treatment at Discharge	1656	Process

[a] Please note that NQF identifies #2020 as a structure measure.
SOURCE: NQF Quality Positioning System (NQF, 2015).

existing clinical data (Byron et al., 2014; Kilbourne et al., 2010; Pincus et al., 2011).

Most of the endorsed measures listed in Table 5-1 are used to evaluate processes of care. Of the 13 outcome measures, 4 are focused on depression. The endorsed measures address care in inpatient and outpatient settings, and several address screening and care coordination. Few address patient-centeredness.

While the NQF endorsement process focuses on performance measures for assessing processes and outcomes of care, measures used for accreditation or certification purposes often articulate expectations for structural capabilities and how those resources are used. However, these structural measures do not currently address in detail the infrastructure needed to implement evidence-based psychosocial interventions. Examples are provided in Table 5-2 for clinical practices and hospitals.

TABLE 5-2 Examples of Structural Measures Addressing Mental Health and Substance Use

Source	Measure	Description
Chinman et al., 2003	Competency Assessment Instrument (CAI), Community Resources Scale	The CAI measures 15 competencies needed to provide high-quality care for those with severe and persistent mental illness. The Community Resources scale on the CAI is defined as "refers clients to local employment, self-help, and other rehabilitation programs" (Chinman et al., 2003).
State of New York	Standards for Health Homes	"The health home provider is accountable for engaging and retaining health home enrollees in care; coordinating and arranging for the provision of services; supporting adherence to treatment recommendations; and monitoring and evaluating a patient's needs, including prevention, wellness, medical, specialist, and behavioral health treatment, care transitions, and social and community services where appropriate through the creation of an individual plan of care" (New York State Health Department, 2012).
NCQA	The Medical Home System Survey (MHSS) (NQF #1909)	The MHSS is used to assess the degree to which an individual primary care practice or provider has in place the structures and processes of an evidence-based patient-centered medical home. The survey comprises six composite measures, each used to assess a particular domain of the patient-centered medical home: Composite 1: Enhance access and continuity Composite 2: Identify and manage patient populations Composite 3: Plan and manage care Composite 4: Provide self-care support and community resources Composite 5: Track and coordinate care Composite 6: Measure and improve performance (NQF, 2011)

continued

TABLE 5-2 Continued

Source	Measure	Description
American Nurses Association	Skill mix (registered nurse [RN], licensed vocational/practical nurse [LVN/LPN], unlicensed assistive personnel [UAP], and contract personnel) (NQF #0204)	NSC-12.1—Percentage of total productive nursing hours worked by RNs (employee and contract) with direct patient care responsibilities by hospital unit
		NSC-12.2—Percentage of total productive nursing hours worked by LPNs/LVNs (employee and contract) with direct patient care responsibilities by hospital unit
		NSC-12.3—Percentage of total productive nursing hours worked by UAP (employee and contract) with direct patient care responsibilities by hospital unit
		NSC-12.4—Percentage of total productive nursing hours worked by contract or agency staff (RNs, LPNs/LVNs, and UAP) with direct patient care responsibilities by hospital unit
		Note that the skill mix of the nursing staff (NSC-12.1, NSC-12.2, and NSC-12.3) represents the proportions of total productive nursing hours by each type of nursing staff (RN, LPN/LVN, and UAP); NSC-12.4 is a separate rate. The measure's focus is the structure of care quality in acute care hospital units (NQF, 2009).

A FRAMEWORK FOR THE DEVELOPMENT OF QUALITY MEASURES FOR PSYCHOSOCIAL INTERVENTIONS

To guide the consideration of opportunities to develop quality measures for psychosocial interventions, the committee built on prior work by Brown and colleagues (2014). The discussion here is organized according to the Donabedian model for measuring quality, which uses the categories of structure, process, and outcomes (Donabedian, 1980). The following sections consider opportunities and challenges for each of these types of measures.

Structure Measures

"Structural components have a propensity to influence the process of care . . . changes in the process of care, including variations in quality, will influence the outcomes of care, broadly defined. Hence, structural effects on outcomes are mediated through process."

—Donabedian, 1980, p. 84

Appropriately developed and applied structure measures form the basis for establishing a systematic framework for quality measurement and improvement. Thus, structure measures are viewed as necessary to ensure that key process concepts of care can actually be implemented in a way that conforms to the evidence base linking those concepts to key outcomes (both the achievement of positive outcomes and the avoidance of negative outcomes). Importantly, structure measures generally indicate the potential for these concepts to be applied effectively and to result in the desired outcomes; they are not used to assess whether these capacities are actually implemented in accordance with existing evidence or whether desired outcomes are achieved. They can, however, be used to assess whether the organization/provider has the capabilities necessary to monitor, improve, and report on the implementation of key processes and achievement of desired outcomes.

Structure measures typically are embodied in requirements for federal programs (e.g., requirements for health plans participating in CMS's Comprehensive Primary Care Initiative [CMS, 2015a]), for independent accreditation programs (such as the Joint Commission's accreditation for hospitals [Joint Commission, 2015]), or for NCQA's recognition program for patient-centered medical homes (NCQA, 2015). Structure measures are applied as well in the accreditation programs for training programs for health care providers (e.g., that of the Accreditation Council for Graduate Medical Education [ACGME]). Certification and credentialing programs also apply what are essentially structure measures for assessing whether individual providers meet standards indicating that they have the knowledge, skills, proficiency, and capacity to provide evidence-based care. Typically, accreditation processes rely on documentation submitted by organizations/ providers, augmented by on-site audits, including consumer or staff interviews. Certification programs also rely on information submitted by providers, as well as written, computer-based, or oral examinations, and, increasingly, on observations of actual practice (including assessment of fidelity to a level of competency). In addition, accreditation programs often include requirements for reporting of processes and outcomes (e.g., the Joint Commission's core measures, reporting under the United Kingdom's Improving Access to Psychological Therapies program).

Opportunities

The committee envisions important opportunities to develop and apply structure measures as part of a systematic, comprehensive, and balanced strategy for enhancing the quality of psychosocial interventions. Structure measures can be used to assess providers' training and capacity to offer evidence-based psychosocial interventions. They provide guidance on infrastructure development and best practices. They support credentialing and payment, thereby allowing purchasers and health plans to select clinics or provider organizations that are equipped to furnish evidence-based psychosocial interventions. Finally, they can support consumers in selecting providers with expertise in interventions specific to their condition or adapted to their cultural expectations (Brown et al., 2014). A framework for leveraging these structural concepts to develop quality measures for psychosocial interventions might include the following:

- Population needs assessment—Determination of the array of services/interventions to be provided based on identification and characterization of the needs of the population served by the organization, including clinical (i.e., general/preventive health, mental health, and substance use) and psychosocial needs and recovery perspectives (see IOM, 2008) (through either direct provision of services or referral arrangements with other providers). Needs assessment can also consider the diversity of the population in terms of race/ethnicity, culture, sexual identity, disability, and other factors that may affect care needs and opportunities to address disparities.

- Adoption of evidence-based practices—Development and use of internal clinical pathways (including standardized assessment of key patient-centered, recovery-oriented clinical outcomes and processes) that are based on guidelines meeting the IOM standards (or other well-established evidence); that conform to a framework for systematic, longitudinal, coordinated, measurement-based, stepped care (i.e., measurement-based care) (Harding et al., 2011); and that provide a menu of available options for the provision of evidence-based psychosocial interventions.

- Health information technology—Utilization of health information technology (including EHRs) with functionalities that include the creation of registries for the implementation of a monitoring and reporting system, for use both at the point of care and for quality improvement and accountability reporting.

- Quality improvement—Establishment of an ongoing, accountable structure/committee and activities for systematically monitoring data related to quality and safety and implementing strategies for improvement. The committee might include substantive representation from the consumer population served, as well as providers and key leaders of the organization.

- Training and credentialing—Establishment of hiring, training, and credentialing policies to ensure that clinicians meet specific standards for fidelity in the delivery of the psychosocial (or other) interventions they provide to consumers. These policies might be augmented by the provision of ongoing case-based supervision of providers.

- Access and outcome measurement—Implementation of policies and procedures to ensure that the array of strategies, systems, and services established in the items above is, in fact, addressing the needs of key populations. For example, consumers might have adequate access to evidence-based interventions through the implementation of policies regarding hours of clinic/clinician availability, maintenance of adequate workforce, monitoring of wait times, and assessment of consumer perspectives. Strategies for enhancing health literacy, utilizing shared decision-making tools, and providing peer support might be implemented.

Implementing this framework would require the development of a set of measures for evaluating each structural concept. The measures noted in Table 5-3 might be part of that set but would not be the sole measures applicable to that concept.

TABLE 5-3 Opportunities for Measuring the Quality of Psychosocial Interventions Using Structure Measures

Measure Concept	Examples of Existing or Proposed Measures Potentially Applicable to This Concept	Data Sources
Capability for delivering evidence-based psychotherapy	Hiring, training, and supervision of staff	Documentation submitted by provider
Capability for measuring outcomes	Presence of registry with functionality for tracking and outcome assessment	Documentation submitted by provider, reports
Infrastructure for quality improvement	Involvement of consumers in quality improvement	On-site audits, including consumer or staff interviews

SOURCE: Adapted from Brown et al., 2014.

Challenges

A number of challenges must be considered in exploiting the opportunities for developing and implementing structure measures described above:

- While there is strong face validity for these concepts, and most of them are key components of evidence-based chronic care models, they have not been formally tested individually or together.
- Resources would be needed to support both the documentation and the verification of structures.
- Clinical organizations providing care for MH/SU disorders have less well developed information systems compared with general health care and also are excluded from the incentive programs in the Health Information Technology for Economic and Clinical Health (HITECH) Act (CMS, 2015b). The costs of developing the health information technology and other capacities necessary to meet the structural criteria discussed above will require additional resources.
- The infrastructure for clinician training, competency assessment, and certification in evidence-based psychosocial interventions is neither well developed nor standardized at the local or national level. For MH/SU clinical organizations to implement their own clinician training and credentialing programs would be highly inefficient.
- Many providers of care for MH/SU disorders work in solo or small practices and lack access to the infrastructure assumed for the concepts discussed above. There would need to be a substantial restructuring of the practice environment and shift of incentives to encourage providers to link with organizations that could provide this infrastructure support. Incentive strategies would need to go beyond those associated with reimbursement (perhaps involving licensure and certification), because a significant proportion of providers of MH/SU care do not accept insurance (Bishop et al., 2014).

Process Measures

"[Measuring the process of care] is justified by the assumption that . . . what is now known to be 'good' medical care has been applied. . . . The estimates of quality that one obtains are less stable and less final than those that derive from the measurement of outcomes. They may,

however, be more relevant to the question at hand: whether medicine is properly practiced."

—*Donabedian, 2005, p. 694*

Ideally, process measures are selected in areas in which scientific studies have established an association between the provision of particular services and the probability of achieving desired outcomes (McGlynn, 1998) through evidence from randomized controlled trials or observational studies. Examples include the association between receipt of guideline-concordant care and better clinical depression outcomes in routine practice settings (Fortney et al., 2001) and the association between engagement in substance abuse treatment and decreased criminal justice involvement (Garnick et al., 2007). Process measures that track access to services or encounters with MH/SU care delivery systems for which evidence for impact on outcomes is lacking may be useful as measures of service utilization or access to care. Process measures that can be captured through existing data from either administrative claims or medical records (e.g., filled prescriptions, lab tests, results of lab tests) have traditionally been appealing because they take advantage of existing data. However, the focus of the field of quality measurement, at least with regard to accountability measures, is shifting to outcomes and eschewing process measures unless they are proximal to outcomes. Process measures, however, remain important for improvement activities.

Opportunities

The committee sees important opportunities to develop and apply process measures as part of a systematic, comprehensive, and balanced strategy for enhancing the quality of psychosocial interventions. Defining the processes of care associated with evidence-based psychosocial interventions is complicated. However, effective and efficient measures focused on the delivery of evidence-based psychosocial interventions are important opportunities for supporting the targeting and application of improvement strategies (Brown et al., 2014), and currently used data sources offer several opportunities to track the processes of care (see Table 5-4):

- Monitoring the delivery of psychosocial interventions as a measure of access to these services—There is growing concern about the underutilization of psychotherapy in the treatment of MH/SU disorders. Tracking the use of psychotherapy through claims data is one approach to monitoring its delivery. Claims data could be used to determine whether psychotherapy was used at all for persons with certain conditions and to better understand patterns of utilization related to timing and duration (Brown et al., 2014). Examples of strategies for assessing access include patient surveys and internal waiting list data. Because patient surveys may not provide immediate feedback on availability of services, approaches for using simulated patients or "mystery shoppers" to contact providers to assess appointment availability have also been used (Steinman et al., 2012).

- Tracking the content of evidence-based psychosocial interventions—Better understanding the content of encounters for MH/SU disorders and whether evidence-based psychosocial interventions are actually provided is essential for tracking the delivery of such interventions.
  - Claims data could be used for this purpose if enhanced procedure codes were developed. More specific procedure codes could be used to capture the content and targets of psychosocial interventions, particularly if aligned with ongoing international and national efforts focused on establishing a common terminology and classification system for psychosocial interventions. These codes could be tied to structure measures related to provider credentialing. Such descriptive billing codes could relate to specific psychotherapeutic processes, and the use of such codes could be restricted to providers who have demonstrated competency, such as through credentialing (Brown et al., 2014).
  - As EHRs become more widely adopted in the delivery of MH/SU services, incorporating structured fields on the content of psychosocial interventions could facilitate better documentation and easier extraction of data for constructing quality measures. Computerized extraction of content information from medical notes is another potential approach (Brown et al., 2014). A common terminology and classification system for psychotherapy could provide the basis for coding and documenting the content of care.
  - Clinical registries are another potential opportunity for tracking care and could enable efficiency in implementation, allow standardized reporting, and support coordination across providers and systems.
- Consumer reports on the content of psychosocial interventions—Information on consumers' experiences with care is collected routinely by health plans and provider organizations. Several existing surveys query consumers about their experiences with the delivery of MH/SU services, although they do not focus on the specific content of psychotherapy. These types of surveys could be used

TABLE 5-4 Opportunities for Measuring the Quality of Psychosocial Interventions Using Process Measures

Measure Concept	Examples of Existing or Proposed Measures	Data Sources
Access/frequency of visits	Psychotherapy visits among people with depression	Claims
Documentation of evidence-based psychosocial interventions	Receipt of adequate number of encounters/content of cognitive-behavioral therapy among people with posttraumatic stress disorder	Medical records or electronic health records
Consumer- and provider-reported content of psychotherapy	Use of peer support among people with schizophrenia; completion of recommended course of psychotherapy	Surveys of patients or providers

SOURCE: Adapted from Brown et al., 2014.

to gather such information. It may also be possible to link this information to clinical outcomes and client satisfaction (Brown et al., 2014). Such measures could give consumers an opportunity to assess the delivery of care and serve as a means of engaging clinicians in discussions about treatment.

- Provider reports on the content of care—Such reports hold some promise. One survey asked providers to rate the frequency with which they delivered each psychotherapy element over the course of treatment (Hepner et al., 2010).

Challenges

A number of challenges need to be considered in the design of process measures, many related to the nature of the data source itself. Claims, EHRs, and consumer surveys all pose challenges as data sources for these measures.

Claims, while readily available, exist for the purpose of payment, not tracking the content of treatment. Procedure codes used for billing lack detail on the content of psychotherapy; the codes have broad labels such as "individual psychotherapy" and "group psychotherapy" (APA, 2013). A further complication is that state Medicaid programs have developed their own psychotherapy billing codes, and these, too, provide no detail on the content of the psychotherapy (Brown et al., 2014). A key issue, discussed in Chapter 3, is the lack of a common terminology for the various components and forms of psychosocial interventions. Such a terminology would need to be instantiated in a standardized intervention classification system like the American Medical Association's (AMA's) Current Procedural Terminology (CPT). The potential harmonization between the AMA CPT codes and the World Health Organization's (WHO's) International Classification of Health Interventions might be an opportunity for developing an approach for more useful coding of psychosocial interventions (Tu et al., 2014).

Still, billing practices vary widely, which poses a challenge to making valid comparisons across providers. Even if appropriate billing codes reflecting content could be developed, it is uncertain whether they would actually be applied in a valid manner without an audit process. As the health care system moves away from fee-for-service payment and toward bundled payment approaches, the use of such codes for billing may become less likely.

Clinical records, including EHRs and registries, have potential to enable tracking of the receipt of evidence-based care, provided that the necessary data elements are available electronically. Clinical data registries also could be useful for tracking the processes and outcomes of care for MH/SU conditions. However, current EHRs and registries do not contain fields capturing psychosocial health or specific psychotherapy content (Glasgow et al., 2012). Detailed information on therapy sessions in EHRs also could pose a threat to confidentiality, and could make confidentiality protection more of a concern for both consumers and providers. More important, the recording of specific psychotherapies or the content of psychotherapy would represent a major change in documentation, and this additional burden might not be well accepted. Efforts to lessen the burden of documentation would have to be weighed against the need to ensure that reports are meaningful. Concern also has been raised about measures that allow providers to "check the box," with little opportunity to verify the content or report.

With respect to consumer surveys, the surveys need to be capable of detecting variations in the delivery of the specific content of psychotherapeutic treatment. However, research on substance use treatment and multisystemic therapy suggests that consumers may not be valid reporters on the content of psychosocial interventions they receive (Chapman et al., 2013; Schoenwald et al., 2009), although data on consumer reports of cognitive-behavioral therapy are promising (Miranda et al., 2010). Consumers may have difficulty recalling therapy sessions, the elements of psychotherapy may change during the course of treatment, and there are burdens and costs associated with data collection (Brown et al., 2014). Finally, consumers may not be interested in providing feedback, making the collection of sufficient information to make reliable comparisons across providers a challenge.

The validity of provider reporting on the content of psychotherapy is not well established. Providers tend to overestimate their delivery of treatment content, especially if a measure is linked to performance appraisals or payment (Schoenwald et al., 2011). Similarly, providers overestimate their ability to follow treatment protocols compared with the assessments of independent raters (Chapman et al., 2013). Another disadvantage is that providers may have difficulty recalling therapy sessions; the best time to query them may be immediately following a session (Brown et al., 2014).

Finally, measures for assessing the delivery of psychosocial interventions would ideally require detailed information on patient characteristics (e.g., diagnosis, severity) and the intervention (e.g., timing, content) to make it possible to determine the degree to which the intervention was implemented in accordance with the clinical trials demonstrating its effectiveness.

Given the above challenges, process measures that address access to services may be ready for implementation in the short term, while those addressing the content of care may require more detailed study and be better suited to supporting quality improvement efforts.

Outcome Measures

"Outcomes do have . . . the advantage of reflecting all contributions to care, including those of the patient. But this advantage is also a handicap, since it is not possible to say precisely what went wrong unless the antecedent process is scrutinized."

—Donabedian, 1988, p. 1746

Of all quality measures, outcome measures have the greatest potential value for patients, families, clinicians, and payers because they indicate whether patients have improved or reached their highest level of function and whether full symptom or disease remission has been achieved. One of the earliest and most widely used conceptual models of health care outcomes, described by Wilson and Cleary (1995), integrates concepts of biomedical patient outcomes and quality-of-life measures. Wilson and Cleary identify five domains that are influenced by characteristics of both the patient and the environment: (1) biological and physiological variables, (2) symptoms, (3) functional status, (4) general health perceptions, and (5) overall quality of life. This model encompasses the interaction and causal linkages among clinical, biological, environmental, and societal variables that influence an individual's health status. Subsequent models of health care outcomes encompass economic dimensions as well, including direct and indirect costs; resource utilization; disability; and outcomes external to the health care system, such as employment, absenteeism, incarceration, and legal charges (Velentgas et al., 2013). Other models add consumer experiences with care (Lebow, 1983; Williams, 1994) and measures reflecting full recovery from mental health disorders (Deegan, 1988; Scheyett et al., 2013).

Patient-reported outcome measures are appealing because they can be used to monitor patient progress, guide clinical decision making, and engage consumers in care. Patient-reported outcomes shift the focus from the content of the intervention to its results; quality measures that evaluate outcomes overcome the limitations of structure and process measures. Outcome measures also offer a means of making care more patient-centered by permitting consumers to report directly on their symptoms and functioning. And the measures provide tangible feedback that consumers can use for self-monitoring and for making treatment decisions.

Importantly, outcome measures can be used to identify patients who are not responding to treatment or may require treatment modifications, as well as to gauge individual provider and system performance and to identify opportunities for quality improvement (Brown et al., 2014).

Patient-reported outcomes are integral to measurement-based care (Harding et al., 2011; Hermann, 2005), which is predicated on the use of brief, standardized, specific assessment measures for target symptoms or behaviors that guide a patient-centered action plan. Without standardized measurement, the provider's appraisal of the patient's symptom remission may result in suboptimal care or only partial remission (Sullivan, 2008). While measurement cannot replace clinical judgment, standardized measurement at each visit or at periodic intervals regarding specific target symptoms informs both provider and patient about relative progress toward symptom resolution and restoration of a full level of function and quality of life. Measurement-based care helps both provider and patient modify and evaluate the plan of care to achieve full symptom remission and support full or the highest level of recovery from an MH/SU disorder.

Opportunities

The committee sees important opportunities to develop and apply quality measures based on patient-reported outcomes as part of a systematic, comprehensive, and balanced strategy for enhancing the quality of psychosocial interventions. Priority domains for these quality measures include symptom reduction/remission functional status, patient/consumer perceptions of care, and recovery outcomes.

Symptom reduction/remission There are a number of examples of widely used, brief, standardized measures for target symptoms. They include the Patient Health Questionnaire (PHQ)-9[1] (Kroenke et al., 2001), Generalized Anxiety Disorder (GAD)-7[2] (Spitzer et al., 2006), and Adult ADHD Self-Report Scale (ASRS) (Wolraich et al., 2003).

Functional status Functional status commonly refers to both the ability to perform and the actual performance of activities or tasks that are important for independent living and crucial to the fulfillment of relevant roles within an individual's life circumstances (IOM, 1991). *Functional ability* refers to an individual's actual or potential capacity to perform activities and tasks that one normally expects of an adult (IOM, 1991). *Functional status* refers to an individual's actual performance of activities and tasks associated with current life roles (IOM, 1991). There exist a variety of functional assessment measures tailored for different populations or for condition-specific assessments using different functional domains of health. Examples include the Older Americans Resources and Services (OARS) scale (Fillenbaum and Smyer, 1981), the Functional Assessment Rating Scale (FARS) (Ward et al., 2006), and the 36-Item Short Form Health Survey (SF-36) (McDowell, 2006; Ware, 2014). For measurement of general health, well-being, and level of function, a variety of tools are available, including both the SF-36, a proprietary instrument with similar public domain versions (RAND 36-Item Health Survey [RAND-36], Veterans RAND 12-Item Health Survey [VR-12]), and the Patient Reported Outcomes Measurement Information System (PROMIS) tools (NIH, 2014). The PROMIS tools, developed through research funded by the National Institutes of Health (NIH) and in the public domain, are garnering interest because they are psychometrically sound and address key domains of physical, mental, and social functioning (Bevans et al., 2014).

When selecting functional assessment measures, one needs to be mindful of their intended use, value for clinical assessment or research, established validity and reliability, and floor and ceiling effects. This last consideration is important when evaluating functional ability in patients who may be at their highest level of the measure with little to no variability; patients at the lowest level of functioning will likewise have little variability. Change in function may not be feasible in many chronic disorders, with maintenance of functional status or prevention of further decline being the optimal possible outcome (Richmond et al., 2004).

---

[1] Patient Health Questionnaire (PHQ) Screeners. See http://phqscreeners.com/pdfs/02_PHQ-9/English.pdf (accessed June 22, 2015).

[2] Patient Health Questionnaire (PHQ) Screeners. See http://www.phqscreeners.com/pdfs/03_GAD-7/English.pdf (accessed June 22, 2015).

Patient/consumer perceptions of care Information on patients' perceptions of care enables comparisons across providers, programs, and facilities, and can help identify gaps in service quality across systems and promote effective quality improvement strategies. Dimensions of patient perceptions of care include (1) access to care, (2) shared decision making, (3) communication, (4) respect for the individual and other aspects of culturally and linguistically appropriate care, and (5) overall ratings and willingness to recommend to others. The most widely used tools for assessing patient experiences of care include the Consumer Assessment of Healthcare Providers and Services (CAHPS) instruments for hospitals, health plans, and providers, as well as the Experience of Care and Health Outcomes (ECHO) survey, which is used to assess care in behavioral health settings (AHRQ, 2015a,b). The Mental Health Statistics Improvement Program (MHSIP) is a model consumer survey initiated in 1976 with state and federal funding (from HHS) to support the development of data standards for evaluating public mental health systems. It has evolved over the past 38 years, and the University of Washington now conducts the 32-item online Adult Consumer Satisfaction Survey (ACS) and the 26-item Youth and Family Satisfaction Survey (YFS). These two surveys are used to assess general satisfaction with services, the appropriateness and quality of services, participation in treatment goals, perception of access to services, and perceived outcomes (UW, 2013). These MHSIP surveys, used by 55 states and territories in the United States, provide a "mental health care report card" for consumers, state and federal agencies, legislative bodies, and third-party payers. Positive perceptions of care are associated with higher rates of service utilization and improved outcomes, including health status and health-related quality of life (Anhang Price et al., 2014).

Recovery outcomes Recovery increasingly is recognized as an important outcome, particularly from a consumer perspective. Research shows that people with serious mental illnesses can and do recover from those illnesses (Harding et al., 1987; Harrow et al., 2012). Personal recovery is associated with symptom reduction, fewer psychiatric hospitalizations, and improved residential stability (SAMHSA, 2011). Still, only recently has recovery become an overarching aim of mental health service systems (Slade et al., 2008).

Recovery is viewed as a process of change through which individuals improve their health and wellness, live a self-directed life, and strive to achieve their full potential (SAMHSA, 2011). As Deegan (1988, p. 1) notes, recovery is "to live, work, and love in a community in which one makes a significant contribution." The Substance Abuse and Mental Health Services Administration (SAMHSA) has identified four dimensions that support a life in recovery: (1) health, with an individual making informed health choices that support physical and emotional well-being; (2) home, where an individual has a stable, safe place to live; (3) purpose, with an individual engaging in meaningful daily activities (e.g., job, school, volunteering); and (4) community, wherein an individual builds relationships and social networks that provide support (SAMHSA, 2011).

Measure developers have made different assumptions regarding the underlying mechanisms of recovery and included different domains in their recovery outcome measures (Scheyett et al., 2013). Several instruments—including the Consumer Recovery Outcomes System (Bloom and Miller, 2004), the Recovery Assessment Scale (RAS) (Corrigan et al., 1999; Salzer and Brusilovskiy, 2014), and the Recovery Process Inventory (Jerrell et al., 2006)—have strong psychometric properties. The RAS in particular has been used in the United States with good results. It is based on five domains: (1) confidence/hope, (2) willingness to ask for help, (3) goal and success orientation, (4) reliance on others, and (5) no domination by symptoms (Corrigan et al., 1999; Salzer and Brusilovskiy, 2014).

Quality measures based on patient-reported outcomes It is important to distinguish between the patient-reported outcome measures discussed above and the quality measures that are based on them. Table 5-5 summarizes opportunities for measuring the quality of psychosocial interventions using patient-reported outcome measures. Quality measures based on patient-reported outcome measures typically define a specific population at risk, a time period for observation, and an expected change or improvement in outcome score. For example, the CMS EHR incentive program ("Meaningful Use") includes a quality measure (NQF #710) assessing remission in symptoms among people with a diagnosis of depression or dysthymia at 12 months following a visit with elevated symptoms as scored using the PHQ-9 (CMS, 2015c,d).

Brief patient-reported or clinician-administered scales with sound psychometrics that are in the public domain could be widely adopted by health care providers and agencies. Wide-scale adoption of these scales or their mandated use by payers for reimbursement would advance understanding of best practices that yield optimal clinical outcomes. Another key opportunity is giving MH/SU providers incentives to use standardized clinical outcome reporting through either EHRs or other clinical databases.

Challenges

A number of challenges are entailed in measuring MH/SU outcomes. These involve (1) determination of which measures and which outcomes to use; (2) accountability and the lack of a standardized methodology for risk adjustment related to complexity, risk profile, and comorbidities; (3) the

TABLE 5-5 Opportunities for Measuring the Quality of Psychosocial Interventions Using Outcome Measures

Measure Concept	Examples of Existing Patient-Reported Outcome Measures	Examples of Existing or Potential Quality Measures Using Patient-Reported Outcome Measures
Recovery	Recovery Assessment Scale (RAS)	Consumers with serious and persistent mental illness who improve by x% on the RAS
Patient experiences of care	Experience of Care and Health Outcomes (ECHO), Consumer Assessment of Healthcare Providers and Systems (CAHPS), Mental Health Statistics Improvement Program (MHSIP)	Proportion of clients of mental health clinics who report participation in treatment decision making
Reduction/remission of symptoms	Patient Health Questionnaire (PHQ)-9	Depression remission among patients with major depression and elevated symptom score
Functioning/well-being	36-Item Short Form Health Survey (SF-36), Patient Reported Outcomes Measurement Information System (PROMIS)-29	Improvement in social functioning among consumers enrolled in managed care

SOURCE: Adapted from Brown et al., 2014.

lack of a cohesive and comprehensive plan requiring the use of standardized MH/SU outcome measures as part of routine care; and (4) the difficulty of extracting data and the lack of electronic health information.

Determination of which measures and which outcomes Without a universally accepted set of outcome measures, clinicians and payers cannot readily compare individual patient outcomes, clinician or provider outcomes, agency outcomes, or population-wide outcomes. Few nationally endorsed measures address outcomes of care, and these few measures address only two domains—symptoms and consumer experiences. Among the NQF-endorsed outcome measures are two assessing depression symptom response, two addressing depression symptom remission, and one addressing consumer experiences with behavioral health services.[3] Thus, there exists a

---

[3] See Table 5-1 for information on outcome measures NQF #1884, #1885, #0710, #0711, and #0726.

gap in available outcome measures for the other major MH/SU disorders, as well as for quality of life and full recovery.

The focus on symptom response/remission measures also does not take into account the fact that consumers with an MH/SU disorder often have multiple comorbid conditions. They also rarely receive only one psychosocial intervention, more often receiving a combination of services, such as medication management and one or more psychosocial interventions, making assessment of overall response to MH/SU services appealing. Outcome measures look at overall impact on the consumer and are particularly relevant for psychosocial interventions that have multifactorial, person-centered dimensions.

The large number of tools available for assessing diverse outcomes makes comparisons across organizations and populations highly challenging. In the CMS EHR incentive program, specification of quality measures that use patient-reported outcomes requires specific code sets (CMS, 2015b). Use of measures in the public domain can reduce the burden on health information technology vendors and providers. Consensus on tools for certain topics (e.g., the PHQ-9 for monitoring depression symptoms) allows for relative ease of implementation; however, other tools are preferred for specific populations. An initiative called PROsetta stone is under way to link the PROMIS scales with other measures commonly used to assess patient-reported outcomes (Choi et al., 2012). In addition, efforts to develop a credible national indicator for subjective well-being that reflects "how people experience and evaluate their lives and specific domains and activities in their lives" (NRC, 2013, p. 15) have led to several advances that may be worth considering for quality measurement.

Accountability and the lack of a standardized methodology for risk adjustment Because outcomes can be influenced by myriad factors related to the person's illness, resources, and history as well as treatment, the opportunity for a clinician or organization to influence outcomes may be limited. Determining the appropriate level of accountability for outcome measures is important since health plans or larger entities may have more opportunities for influencing outcomes and because the risk may be spread across a broader population.

Valid risk adjustment plays a critical role in the successful use of outcome measures by making it possible to avoid disincentives to care for the most complex and severely ill patients. Yet while risk adjustment models have been developed for a variety of medical disorders and surgical procedures, they are less well developed for MH/SU disorders (Ettner et al., 1998). A review of the risk adjustment literature identified 36 articles that included 72 models of utilization, 74 models of cost expenditures, and 15 models of clinical outcomes (Hermann et al., 2007). An average of

6.7 percent of the variance in these areas was explained by models using diagnostic and sociodemographic data, while an average of 22.8 percent of the variance was explained by models using more detailed clinical and quality-of-life data (Hermann et al., 2007). Risk adjustment models based on administrative or claims data explained less than one-third of the variance explained by models that included clinical assessment or medical records data (Hermann et al., 2007). Consensus on a reasonable number of clinical outcome and quality indicators is needed among payers, regulators, and behavioral health organizations to enable the development of risk adjustment models that can account for the interactions among different risk factors.

The lack of a cohesive and comprehensive plan requiring the use of standardized MH/SU outcome measures Comprehensive approaches such as the MHSIP could serve as a model for standardizing measures for MH/SU disorders; however, even that program does not extend to outcomes other than consumer satisfaction, nor does it cover individuals or care outside of the public sector. Efforts to encourage the use of outcome measurement need to be carried out at multiple levels and to involve multiple stakeholders. Consumers need to be encouraged to track their own recovery; clinicians to monitor patient responses and alter treatment strategies based on those responses; and organizations to use this information for quality improvement, network management, and accountability.

Difficulty of extracting data and lack of electronic health information Even if a basic set of outcome measures were universally endorsed, the information obtained would remain fragmented absent agencies and payers committed to developing the infrastructure needed to collect the data for the measures. Aggregating valid data on clinical outcomes is a time-consuming and costly endeavor. Currently, electronic health information that links health care across different providers and agencies is lacking. Even in self-contained systems such as a health maintenance organization (HMO), where electronic data entry can be designed for linkages across providers and levels of care within the system, it can be difficult to obtain consistently valid data (Strong et al., 1997).

As with structure and process measures, improved measurement of clinical outcomes will benefit from the universal adoption of EHRs. Universal use of EHRs will make it possible to link health care and health outcomes across different providers and agencies over time, compare clinical outcomes associated with different treatment approaches, and develop risk adjustment models through assessment of a large national dataset.

CONCLUSION AND RECOMMENDATIONS

The Donabedian framework of structure, process, and outcome measures offers an excellent model for developing measures with which to assess the quality of psychosocial interventions. However, few rigorous quality measures are available for assessing whether individuals have access to or benefit from evidence-based psychosocial interventions. The factors contributing to the lack of attention to quality measurement in this area are common to MH/SU disorders in general and point to the same problems identified by the IOM in its report on MH/SU disorders (IOM, 2006). Despite the diverse players in the quality field, strategic leadership and responsibility are lacking for MH/SU care quality in general and for psychosocial interventions in particular. Furthermore, the involvement of consumers in the development and implementation of quality measures is limited in the MH/SU arena.

Systems for accountability and improvement need to focus on improving outcomes for individuals regardless of modality of treatment, yet the infrastructure for measurement and improvement of psychosocial interventions (at both the national level for measure development and the local level for measure implementation and reporting) is lacking. As a result of the lack of standardized reporting of clinical detail and variations in coding, the most widely used data systems for quality reporting fail to capture critical information needed for assessing psychosocial interventions (IOM, 2014). There has as yet been no strategic leadership to harness the potential for addressing this gap through the nation's historic investment in health information technology.

Current quality measures are insufficient to drive improvement in psychosocial interventions. NCQA's annual report on health care quality in managed care plans highlights the lack of improvement in several existing MH/SU quality measures and declining performance for other measures, some of which are summarized in Table 5-6 (NCQA, 2014). While there is enthusiasm for incorporating quality measures based on patient-reported outcome measures, there is no consensus on which outcomes should take priority and what tools are practical and feasible for use in guiding ongoing clinical care, as well as monitoring the performance of the health care system, with respect to treatment for MH/SU disorders.

The entity designated by HHS to assume this responsibility and leadership role needs to ensure coordination among all relevant agencies across the federal government—such as CMS, SAMHSA, the National Institute on Drug Abuse (NIDA), the National Institute of Mental Health (NIMH), the National Institute on Alcohol Abuse and Alcoholism (NIAAA), the Agency for Healthcare Research and Quality (AHRQ), the Health Resources and Services Administration (HRSA), the U.S. Department of Veterans Affairs

TABLE 5-6 Examples of Structure, Process, and Outcome Measures

Example Psychosocial Intervention	Structure	Process	Outcome
Assertive Community Treatment	Care manager training and caseload	Fidelity assessment using Dartmouth Assertive Community Treatment Scale (DACTS) instrument	Percentage of patients with housing instability at initiation of treatment who are in stable housing at 6 months
Cognitive-Behavioral Therapy	Clinicians certified through competency-based training and assessment	Fidelity assessed through electronic health record documentation and periodic review of audiotaped sessions using a standardized assessment tool	Percentage of patients with depression who are in remission at 6 months as assessed by the Patient Health Questionnaire (PHQ)-9

(VA), and the U.S. Department of Defense (DoD)—in order to make sufficient resources available and avoid duplication of effort. Also essential is coordination with relevant nongovernmental organizations, such as NQF, NCQA, and the Patient-Centered Outcomes Research Institute (PCORI), as well professional associations and private payers, to support widespread adoption of the measures developed in multipayer efforts. The designated entity needs to be responsible for using a multistakeholder process to develop strategies for identifying measure gaps, establishing priorities for measure development, and determining mechanisms for evaluating the impact of measurement activities. In these efforts, representation and consideration of the multiple disciplines involved in the delivery of behavioral health care treatment are essential. Consumer/family involvement needs to encompass participation in multistakeholder panels that guide measure development; efforts to garner broad input, such as focus groups; and specific efforts to obtain input on how to present the findings of quality measurement in ways that are meaningful to consumers/families.

In the short term, structure measures that set expectations for the infrastructure needed to support outcome measurement and the delivery of evidence-based psychosocial interventions need to be a priority to establish the capacity for the expanded routine clinical use of outcome measures. A second priority is the development of process measures that can be used to assess access to care (in light of concerns about expanded populations with access to MH/SU care under the ACA and the limited availability of specialty care and evidence-based services). Other process measures addressing the content of care can be used for hypothesis generation and testing with regard to quality improvement. The measurement strategy needs to take into account how performance measures can be used to support patient care in real time, as well as the quality improvement efforts of care teams, organizations, plans, and states, and to encompass efforts to assess the impact of policies concerning the application of quality measures at the local, state, and federal levels. HHS is best positioned to lead efforts to gain consensus on the priority of developing and applying patient-reported outcome measures for use in quality assessment and of validating patient-reported outcome measures for gap areas such as recovery. Standardized and validated patient-reported outcome measures are necessary for performance measurement.

The committee drew the following conclusion about the development of approaches to measure quality of psychosocial interventions:

Approaches applied in other areas of health care can be applied in care for mental health and substance use disorders to develop reliable, valid, and feasible quality measures for both improvement and accountability purposes.

Recommendation 5-1. *Conduct research to contribute to the development, validation, and application of quality measures.* Federal, state, and private research funders and payers should establish a coordinated effort to invest in research to develop measures for assessing the structure, process, and outcomes of care, giving priority to

- measurement of access and outcomes;
- development and testing of quality measures, encompassing patient-reported outcomes in combination with clinical decision support and clinical workflow improvements;
- evaluation and improvement of the reliability and validity of measures;
- processes to capture key data that could be used for risk stratification or adjustment (e.g., severity, social support, housing);
- attention to documentation of treatment adjustment (e.g., what steps are taken when patients are not improving); and
- establishment of structures that support monitoring and improvement.

Recommendation 5-2. *Develop and continuously update a portfolio of measures with which to assess the structure, process, and outcomes of care.* The U.S. Department of Health and Human Services (HHS) should designate a locus of responsibility and leadership for the development of quality measures related to mental health and substance use disorders, with particular emphasis on filling the gaps in measures that address psychosocial interventions. HHS should support and promote the development of a balanced portfolio of measures for assessing the structure, process, and outcomes of care, giving priority to measuring access and outcomes and establishing structures that support the monitoring and improvement of access and outcomes.

Recommendation 5-3. *Support the use of health information technology for quality measurement and improvement of psychosocial interventions.* Federal, state, and private payers should support investments in the development of new and the improvement of existing data and coding systems to support quality measurement and improvement of psychosocial interventions. Specific efforts are needed to encourage broader use of health information technology and the development of data systems for tracking individuals' care and its outcomes over time and across settings. Registries used in other specialty care, such as bariatric treatment, could serve as a model. In addition, the U.S. Department of Health and Human Services should lead efforts involving organizations responsible for coding systems to improve standard code sets for electronic and administrative data (such as Current Procedural Terminology [CPT] and Systematized Nomenclature of Medicine [SNOMED]) to allow the capture of process and outcome data needed to evaluate mental health/substance use care in general and psychosocial interventions in particular. This effort will be facilitated by the identification of the elements of psychosocial interventions and development of a common terminology as proposed under Recommendation 3-1. Electronic and administrative data should include methods for coding disorder severity and other confounding and mitigating factors to enable the development and application of risk adjustment approaches, as well as methods for documenting the use of evidence-based treatment approaches.

REFERENCES

AHRQ (Agency for Healthcare Research and Quality). 2010. *National healthcare disparities report.* http://www.ahrq.gov/research/findings/nhqrdr/nhdr11/nhdr11.pdf (accessed February 17, 2015).
_____. 2015a. *CAHPS surveys and tools to advance patient-centered care.* https://cahps.ahrq.gov (accessed June 15, 2015).
_____. 2015b. *Experience of Care and Health Outcomes (ECHO).* https://www.cahps.ahrq.gov/surveys-guidance/echo/index.html (accessed June 15, 2015).

Anhang Price, R., M. N. Elliott, A. M. Zaslavsky, R. D. Hays, W. G. Lehrman, L. Rybowski, S. Edgman-Levitan, and P. D. Cleary. 2014. Examining the role of patient experience surveys in measuring health care quality. *Medical Care Research and Review* 71(5):522-554.

APA (American Psychological Association). 2013. *Psychotherapy CPT codes for psychologists.* http://www.apapracticecentral.org/reimbursement/billing/psychotherapy-codes.pdf (accessed January 28, 2015).

Bevans, M., A. Ross, and D. Cella. 2014. Patient-Reported Outcomes Measurement Information System (PROMIS): Efficient, standardized tools to measure self-reported health and quality of life. *Nursing Outlook* 62(5):339-345.

Bishop, T. F., M. J. Press, S. Keyhani, and H. A. Pincus. 2014. Acceptance of insurance by psychiatrists and the implications for access to mental health care. *JAMA Psychiatry* 71(2):176-181.

Bloom, B. L., and A. Miller. 2004. *The Consumer Recovery Outcomes System (CROS 3.0): Assessing clinical status and progress in persons with severe and persistent mental illness.* http://www.crosllc.com/CROS3.0manuscript-090204.pdf (accessed December 15, 2014).

Brown, J., S. H. Scholle, and M. Azur. 2014. *Strategies for measuring the quality of psychotherapy: A white paper to inform measure development and implementation.* Report submitted to the Assistant Secretary for Planning and Evaluation, U.S. Department of Health and Human Services. Contract number HHSP23320095642WC and task order number HHSP 23320100019WI. Washington, DC: Mathematica Policy Research. http://aspe.hhs.gov/daltcp/reports/2014/QualPsy.cfm (accessed July 20, 2015).

Burstin, H. 2014. *Issues in quality measurement: The NQF perspective.* Presentation to Committee on Developing Evidence-Based Standards for Psychosocial Interventions for Mental Disorders. Workshop on Approaches to Quality Measurement, May 19, Washington, DC. http://iom.edu/~/media/Files/ActivityFiles/MentalHealth/PsychosocialInterventions/WSI/HelenBurstin.pdf (accessed December 18, 2014).

Byron, S. C., W. Gardner, L. C. Kleinman, R. Mangione-Smith, J. Moon, R. Sachdeva, M. A. Schuster, G. L. Freed, G. Smith, and S. H. Scholle. 2014. Developing measures for pediatric quality: Methods and experiences of the CHIPRA pediatric quality measures program grantee. *Academic Pediatrics* 14(5):S27-S32. Reprinted with permission from Elsevier.

Chapman, J. E., M. R. McCart, E. J. Letourneau, and A. J. Sheidow. 2013. Comparison of youth, caregiver, therapist, trained, and treatment expert raters of therapist adherence to a substance abuse treatment protocol. *Journal of Consulting and Clinical Psychology* 81(4):674-680.

Chinman, M., A. S. Young, M. Rowe, S. Forquer, E. Knight, and A. Miller. 2003. An instrument to assess competencies of providers treating severe mental illness. *Mental Health Services Research* 5(2):97-108.

Choi, S. W., T. Podrabsky, N. McKinney, B. D. Schalet, K. F. Cook, and D. Cella. 2012. *PROSetta Stone™ analysis report: A Rosetta Stone for patient-reported outcomes.* Vol. 1. Chicago, IL: Department of Medical Social Sciences, Feinberg School of Medicine, Northwestern University. http://www.prosettastone.org/Pages/default.aspx (accessed June 16, 2015).

CMS (Centers for Medicare & Medicaid Services). 2015a. *Comprehensive primary care initiative eCQM user manual—Version 4.* http://innovation.cms.gov/Files/x/cpci-ecqm-manual.pdf (accessed June 12, 2015).

———. 2015b. *An introduction to the Medicare EHR Incentive Program for eligible professionals.* https://www.cms.gov/Regulations-and-Guidance/Legislation/EHRIncentivePrograms/downloads/Beginners_Guide.pdf (accessed June 15, 2015).

———. 2015c. *Measure: Depression remission at twelve months.* https://ecqi.healthit.gov/ep/2014-measures-2015-update/depression-remission-twelve-months (accessed June 15, 2015).

_____. 2015d. *Annual update of 2014 eligible hospitals and eligible professionals Electronic Clinical Quality Measures (eCQMs).* http://www.cms.gov/Regulations-and-Guidance/Legislation/EHRIncentivePrograms/Downloads/eCQM_TechNotes2015.pdf (accessed June 15, 2015).

_____. n.d. *CMS measures management system blueprint (the Blueprint) v 11.0.* http://www.cms.gov/Medicare/Quality-Initiatives-Patient-Assessment-Instruments/MMS/MeasuresManagementSystemBlueprint.html (accessed October 1, 2014).

Conway, P. H., and C. Clancy. 2009. Transformation of health care at the front line. *Journal of the American Medical Association* 301(7):763-765.

Corrigan, P. W., D. Giffort, F. Rashid, M. Leary, and I. Okeke. 1999. Recovery as a psychological construct. *Community Mental Health Journal* 35(3):231-239.

Deegan, P. E. 1988. Recovery: The lived experience of rehabilitation. *Journal of Psychosocial Rehabilitation* 11(4):11-19.

Donabedian, A. 1980. *Explorations in quality assessment and monitoring.* Vol. I. Ann Arbor, MI: Health Administration Press.

_____. 1988. The quality of care. How can it be assessed? *Journal of the American Medical Association* 260(12):1743-1748.

_____. 2005. Evaluating the quality of medical care. 1966. *Milbank Quarterly* 83(4):691-729.

Ettner, S. L., R. G. Frank, T. G. McGuire, J. P. Newhouse, and E. H. Notman. 1998. Risk adjustment of mental health and substance abuse payments. *Inquiry* 35(2):223-239.

Fillenbaum, G. G., and M. A. Smyer. 1981. The development, validity, and reliability of the OARS multidimensional functional assessment questionnaire. *Journal of Gerontology* 36(4):428-434.

Fisher, C. E., B. Spaeth-Rublee, and H. A. Pincus. 2013. Developing mental health-care quality indicators: Toward a common framework. *International Journal for Quality in Health Care* 25(1):75-80.

Fortney, J., K. Rost, M. Zhang, and J. Pyne. 2001. The relationship between quality and outcomes in routine depression care. *Psychiatric Services* 52(1):56-62.

Frank, R. 2014. Presentation to Committee on Developing Evidence-Based Standards for Psychosocial Interventions for Mental Disorders. Workshop on Approaches to Quality Improvement, July 24, Washington, DC.

Garnick, D. W., C. M. Horgan, M. T. Lee, L. Panas, G. A. Ritter, S. Davis, T. Leeper, R. Moore, and M. Reynolds. 2007. Are Washington Circle performance measures associated with decreased criminal activity following treatment? *Journal of Substance Abuse Treatment* 33(4):341-352.

Glasgow, R. E., R. M. Kaplan, J. K. Ockene, E. B. Fisher, and K. M. Emmons. 2012. Patient-reported measures of psychosocial issues and health behavior should be added to electronic health records. *Health Affairs (Millwood)* 31(3):497-504.

Harding, C. M., G. W. Brooks, T. Ashikaga, J. S. Strauss, and A. Breier. 1987. The Vermont longitudinal study of persons with severe mental illness. II: Long-term outcome of subjects who retrospectively met DSM-III criteria for schizophrenia. *American Journal of Psychiatry* 144(6):727-735.

Harding, K. J., A. J. Rush, M. Arbuckle, M. H. Trivedi, and H. A. Pincus. 2011. Measurement-based care in psychiatric practice: A policy framework for implementation. *Journal of Clinical Psychiatry* 72(8):1136-1143.

Harrow, M., T. H. Jobe, and R. N. Faull. 2012. Do all schizophrenia patients need antipsychotic treatment continuously throughout their lifetime? A 20-year longitudinal study. *Psychological Medicine* 42(10):2145-2155.

Hepner, K. A., F. Azocar, G. L. Greenwood, J. Miranda, and M. A. Burnam. 2010. Development of a clinician report measure to assess psychotherapy for depression in usual care settings. *Administration and Policy in Mental Health* 37(3):221-229.

Hermann, R. C. 2005. *Improving mental healthcare: A guide to measurement-based quality improvement.* Washington, DC: American Psychiatric Press, Inc.

Hermann, R. C., C. K. Rollins, and J. A. Chan. 2007. Risk-adjusting outcomes of mental health and substance-related care: A review of the literature. *Harvard Review of Psychiatry* 15(2):52-69.

IOM (Institute of Medicine). 1990. *Medicare: A strategy for quality assurance.* Vol. 1, edited by K. N. Lohr. Washington, DC: National Academy Press.

_____. 1991. Disability concepts revisited: Implications for prevention. In *Disability in America: Toward a national agenda for prevention*, edited by A. M. Pope and A. R. Tarlov. Washington, DC: National Academy Press. Pp. 309-327.

_____. 2006. *Improving the quality of care for mental and substance use conditions.* Washington, DC: The National Academies Press.

_____. 2008. *Cancer care for the whole patient: Meeting psychological health needs.* Washington, DC: The National Academies Press.

_____. 2014. *Capturing social and behavioral domains and measures in electronic health records: Phase 2.* Washington, DC: The National Academies Press.

Jerrell, J. M., V. C. Cousins, and K. M. Roberts. 2006. Psychometrics of the recovery process inventory. *Journal of Behavioral Health Services & Research* 33(4):464-473.

Joint Commission. 2015. *Hospital accreditation.* http://www.jointcommission.org/accreditation/hospitals.aspx (accessed June 12, 2015).

Kilbourne, A., D. Keyser, and H. A. Pincus. 2010. Challenges and opportunities in measuring the quality of mental health care. *Canadian Journal of Psychiatry* 55(9):549-557.

Kroenke, K., R. L. Spitzer, and J. B. W. Williams. 2001. The PHQ-9: Validity of a brief depression severity measure. *Journal of General Internal Medicine* 16(9):606-613.

Lebow, J. L. 1983. Research assessing consumer satisfaction with mental health treatment: A review of findings. *Evaluation and Program Planning* 6:211-236.

Ling, S. M. 2014. *Broad issues in quality measurement: The CMS perspective.* Presentation to Committee on Developing Evidence-Based Standards for Psychosocial Interventions for Mental Disorders. Workshop on Approaches to Quality Measurement, May 19, Washington, DC. https://www.iom.edu/~/media/Files/Activity%20Files/MentalHealth/PsychosocialInterventions/WSI/Shari%20Ling.pdf (accessed December 18, 2014).

McDowell, I. 2006. *Measuring health: A guide to rating scales and questionnaires*, 3rd ed. New York: Oxford University Press

McGlynn, E. A. 1998. Choosing and evaluating clinical performance measures. *Joint Commission Journal on Quality Improvement* 24(9):470-479.

Miranda, J., K. A. Hepner, F. Azocar, G. Greenwood, V. Ngo, and M. A. Burnam. 2010. Development of a patient-report measure of psychotherapy for depression. *Administration and Policy in Mental Health and Mental Health Services Research* 37(3):245-253.

NCQA (National Committee for Quality Assurance). 2014. *State of health care.* http://www.ncqa.org/ReportCards/HealthPlans/StateofHealthCareQuality.aspx (accessed June 15, 2015).

_____. 2015. *Patient-centered medical home recognition.* http://www.ncqa.org/Programs/Recognition/Practices/PatientCenteredMedicalHomePCMH.aspx (accessed June 15, 2015).

New York State Department of Health. 2012. *NYS health home provider qualification standards for chronic medical and behavioral health patient populations.* https://www.health.ny.gov/health_care/medicaid/program/medicaid_health_homes/provider_qualification_standards.htm (accessed January 27, 2015).

NIH (National Institutes of Health). 2014. *PROMIS overview.* http://www.nihpromis.org/about/overview (accessed January 28, 2015).

NQF (National Quality Forum). 2009. *Nursing staff skill mix.* NQF #0204. http://www.qualityforum.org/QPS/0204 (accessed January 27, 2015).
_____. 2011. *Medical Home System Survey (MHSS).* NQF #1909. http://www.qualityforum.org/QPS/1909 (accessed January 27, 2015).
_____. 2014a. *Consensus development process.* http://www.qualityforum.org/Measuring_Performance/Consensus_Development_Process.aspx (accessed April 15, 2015).
_____. 2014b. *Measure applications partnership.* http://www.qualityforum.org/map (accessed January 27, 2015).
_____. 2014c. *Measure evaluation criteria.* http://www.qualityforum.org/docs/measure_evaluation_criteria.aspx (accessed April 27, 2015).
_____. 2015. *Quality positioning system.* http://www.qualityforum.org/QPS/QPSTool.aspx (accessed June 15, 2015).
NQMC (National Quality Measure Clearinghouse). 2014. *Tutorials on quality measures: Desirable attributes of a quality measure.* http://www.qualitymeasures.ahrq.gov (accessed November 6, 2014).
NRC (National Research Council). 2013. *Subjective well-being: Measuring happiness, suffering, and other dimensions of experience.* Washington, DC: The National Academies Press.
Pincus, H. A., B. Spaeth-Rublee, and K. E. Watkins. 2011. Analysis & commentary: The case for measuring quality in mental health and substance abuse care. *Health Affairs (Millwood)* 30(4):730-736.
Richmond, T., S. T. Tang, L. Tulman, J. Fawcett, and R. McCorkle. 2004. Measuring function. In *Instruments for clinical health-care research,* 3rd ed., edited by M. Frank-Stromborg and S. J. Olsen. Sudbury, MA: Jones & Barlett. Pp. 83-99.
Salzer, M. S., and E. Brusilovskiy. 2014. Advancing recovery science: Reliability and validity properties of the Recovery Assessment Scale. *Psychiatric Services* 65(4):442-453.
SAMHSA (Substance Abuse and Mental Health Services Administration). 2011. *SAMHSA's working definition of recovery.* https://store.samhsa.gov/shin/content/PEP12-RECDEF/PEP12-RECDEF.pdf (accessed January 8, 2015).
Scheyett, A., J. DeLuca, and C. Morgan. 2013. Recovery in severe mental illnesses: A literature review of recovery measures. *Social Work Research* 37(3):286-303.
Schoenwald, S. K., J. E. Chapman, A. J. Sheidow, and R. E. Carter. 2009. Long-term youth criminal outcomes in MST transport: The impact of therapist adherence and organizational climate and structure. *Journal of Clinical Child & Adolescent Psychology* 38(1):91-105.
Schoenwald, S. K., A. F. Garland, M. A. Southam-Gerow, B. F. Chorpita, and J. E. Chapman. 2011. Adherence measurement in treatments for disruptive behavior disorders: Pursuing clear vision through varied lenses. *Clinical Psychology (New York)* 18(4):331-341.
Slade, M., M. Amering, and L. Oades. 2008. Recovery: An international perspective. *Epidemiologia e Psichiatria Sociale* 17(2):128-137.
Spitzer, R. L., K. Kroenke, J. B. W. Williams, and B. Löwe. 2006. A brief measure for assessing generalized anxiety disorder: The GAD-7. *Archives of Internal Medicine* 166(10):1092-1097.
Steinman, K. J., K. Kelleher, A. E. Dembe, T. M. Wickizer, and T. Hemming. 2012. The use of a "mystery shopper" methodology to evaluate children's access to psychiatric services. *Journal of Behavioral Health Services & Research* 39(3):305-313.
Strong, D. M., Y. W. Lee, and R. Y. Wang. 1997. Data quality in context. *Communications of the ACM* 40(5):103-110.
Sullivan, G. 2008. Complacent care and the quality gap. *Psychiatric Services* 59(12):1367-1367.

Tu, S. W., C. Nyulas, M. Tierney, A. Syed, R. Musacchio, and T. B. Üstün. 2014. *A content model for health interventions*. Presented at WHO—Family of International Classifications Network Annual Meeting 2014, October 11-17, Barcelona, Spain.

UW (University of Washington). 2013. *Mental Health Statistics Improvement Program (MHSIP) surveys*. Seattle, WA: University of Washington Department of Psychiatry and Behavioral Sciences, Public Behavioral Health and Justice Policy. https://depts.washington.edu/pbhjp/projects-programs/page/mental-health-statistics-improvement-program-adult-consumer-survey-acs (accessed June 15, 2015).

Velentgas, P., N. A. Dreyer, and A. W. Wu. 2013. Outcome definition and measurement. In *Developing a protocol for observational comparative effectiveness research: A user's guide,* Ch. 6, edited by P. Velentgas, N. A. Dreyer, P. Nourjah, S. R. Smith, and M. M. Torchia. Rockville, MD: AHRQ. Pp. 71-92.

Vinik, A. I., and E. Vinik. 2003. Prevention of the complications of diabetes. *American Journal of Managed Care* 9(Suppl. 3):S63-S80; quiz S81-S84.

Ward, J. C., M. G. Dow, K. Penner, T. Saunders, and S. Halls. 2006. *Manual for using the Functional Assessment Rating Scale (FARS)*. http://outcomes.fmhi.usf.edu/FARSUserManual2006.pdf (accessed September 26, 2014).

Ware, J. E. 2014. *SF-36 health survey update*. http://www.sf-36.org/tools/sf36.shtml (accessed January 28, 2015).

Williams, B. 1994. Patient satisfaction: A valid concept? *Social Science and Medicine* 38:509-516.

Wilson, I. B., and P. D. Cleary. 1995. Linking clinical variables with health-related quality of life. A conceptual model of patient outcomes. *Journal of the American Medical Association* 273:59-65.

Wolraich, M. L., W. Lambert, M. A. Doffing, L. Bickman, T. Simmons, and K. Worley. 2003. Psychometric properties of the Vanderbilt ADHD diagnostic parent rating scale in a referred population. *Journal of Pediatric Psychology* 28(8):559-568.

6

Quality Improvement

Previous chapters have addressed the quality of psychosocial interventions in terms of the various types, their efficacy, the potential elements they contain, approaches for assessing the efficacy of these interventions and their elements, the effectiveness of the interventions in actual clinical settings, and the development of guidelines and quality measures to influence and monitor clinical practice. However, these considerations are by themselves insufficient to improve quality. As noted in the Institute of Medicine's (IOM's) Quality Chasm report addressing mental health and substance use conditions (IOM, 2006), a comprehensive quality framework must consider properties beyond the interventions delivered; it must consider the context in which they are delivered. This context includes characteristics of the consumer, the qualifications of the provider, the clinic or specific setting in which care is rendered, the health system or organization in which the setting is embedded, and the regulatory and financial conditions under which it operates. Stakeholders in each of these areas can manipulate levers that shape the quality of a psychosocial intervention; shortfalls in the context of an intervention and in the manipulation of those levers can render a highly efficacious intervention unhelpful or even harmful (for example, levers, see Table 6-1).

Evidence-based psychosocial interventions and meaningful measurement tools are key drivers of quality improvement in the delivery of services for persons with mental health and substance use disorders; however, they will not lead to improvements in quality unless they are used appropriately and applied in a system or organization that is equipped to implement change. This chapter examines the array of levers that can be used by various categories of stakeholders to enhance the quality improvement of psychosocial interventions. The discussion is based on the premise that engaging the perspectives and leveraging the opportunities of multiple stakeholders can best accomplish overall system improvement.

The chapter is organized around five categories of stakeholders:

- *Consumers*—Whether called consumers, clients, or patients, these are the people for whose benefit psychosocial interventions are intended. Consumers and their family members have much to say about and contribute to what these interventions look like and when and how they are used. Indeed, as discussed in earlier chapters, there is growing evidence of consumers' value as active participants in the development, quality measurement, and quality monitoring of psychosocial interventions, as well as in shared decision making in their own recovery process.
- *Providers*—The term is used broadly to include clinicians, rehabilitation counselors, community-based agents who intervene on behalf of individuals in need of psychosocial interventions, peer specialists, and any other professionals who deliver these interventions.
- *Clinical settings/provider organizations*—This term is used broadly to include clinics, practices, large health systems, medical homes, community settings, schools, jails, and other sites where psychosocial interventions are rendered. In clinical settings, quality and quality improvement are affected by some of the same factors as those that affect clinicians, but also by the practice culture, the adequacy of team-based care, clinic workflow, leadership for change and quality improvement, and clinic-level implementation efforts.
- *Health plans and purchasers*—These stakeholders (both public and private) work at the supraclinical level, structuring provider payment, provider networks, benefit design, and utilization management.
- *Regulators*—These include organizations that accredit, certify, and license providers of behavioral health services, including psychosocial interventions. This category can also include organizational regulators, which can ensure that programs are producing clinicians capable of rendering high-quality interventions or that clinics are organized to optimize and ensure the quality of the care delivered.

The levers available to each of these categories of stakeholders are summarized in Table 6-1 and discussed in detail in the following sections. A growing body of research shows the need for deliberate and strategic efforts

TABLE 6-1 Stakeholders and Their Levers for Influencing the Quality of Care for Mental Health and Substance Use Disorders

Stakeholder	Levers for Influencing Quality of Care	Examples
Consumers	• Evaluation • Service provision • Participation in governance • Shared decision making	• Participation/leadership in evaluation • Participation in surveys • Serving as administrators, members of advisory boards • Serving as peer support specialists
Providers	• Postgraduate education • Measurement-based care • Population management • Quality improvement teams • Quality measurement and reporting	• U.K. Improving Access to Psychological Therapies (IAPT) program • Outcome assessment • Tracking outcomes for the practice as a whole, for the population served • U.S. Department of Veterans Affairs (VA) Community of Practice • Dashboards available to clinicians
Clinical Settings/ Provider Organizations	• Care management/ population management/care delivery • Quality improvement infrastructure • Measure reporting and feedback • Electronic data systems • Learning collaboratives • Continuing professional education	• Use of registries • Allowance for team huddles, team-building exercises • Provision of on-site care managers • Shared medical records across disciplines and sites of service • Telehealth resources • Plan, Do, Study, Act teams established and supported
Health Plans/ Purchasers	• Benefit design • Provider network • Provider payment methods • Care management/ coordination • Utilization management	• Pay for performance • Public reporting • Prior authorization requirements • Coinsurance • Value-based insurance design
Regulators	• Accreditation • Licensure	• Training in evidence-based practices • Implementation of evidence-based practices

on the part of all of these stakeholders to ensure that evidence-based psychosocial interventions are adopted, sustained, and delivered effectively in a variety of service delivery settings (Powell et al., 2012; Proctor et al., 2009).

CONSUMERS

Substantive consumer participation—the formal involvement of consumers in the design, implementation, and evaluation of interventions—is known to improve the outcomes of psychosocial interventions (Delman, 2007; Taylor et al., 2009). The unique experience and perspective of consumers also make their active involvement essential to quality management and improvement for psychosocial interventions (Linhorst et al., 2005). To be meaningful, the participation must be sustained over time and focused on crucial elements of the program (Barbato et al., 2014). Roles for consumers include involvement in evaluation, training, management, and service provision, as well as active participation in their own care, such as through shared decision making, self-management programs, and patient-centered medical homes. As noted in Chapter 2, participatory action research (PAR) methods engage consumers. The PAR process necessarily includes resources and training for consumer participants and cross-training among stakeholders (Delman and Lincoln, 2009).

Evaluation

Evidence supports the important role of consumers in program evaluation (Barbato et al., 2014; Drake et al., 2010; Hibbard, 2013). Consumers have been involved at all levels of evaluation, from evaluation design to data collection (Delman, 2007). At the design level, consumer participation helps organizations understand clients' views and expectations for mental health care (Linhorst and Eckert, 2002), and ensures that outcomes meaningful to consumers are included in evaluations and that data are collected in a way that is acceptable to and understood by consumers (Barbato et al., 2014). Further, Clark and colleagues (1999) found that mental health consumers often feel free to talk openly to consumer interviewers, thus providing more honest and in-depth data than can otherwise be obtained. Personal interviews maximize consumer response rates overall and in populations frequently excluded from evaluation (e.g., homeless persons) (Barbato et al., 2014).

Training

Consumers can be valuable members of the workforce training team. The active involvement of consumers in the education and training of health care professionals has been increasing largely because of recognition that patients have unique expertise derived from their experience of illness, treatment, and related socioeconomic detriments (Towle et al., 2010). Consumer participation in clinician training has led to trainees having a more positive attitude toward people with severe mental illness, valuing them as a knowledge resource, reconsidering stereotypes and assumptions about consumers, and improving their communication skills (Taylor et al., 2009; Towle and Godolphin, 2013; Turnbull et al., 2013). Likewise, training has been shown to be effective when consumers play a significant role in developing the format and content of the training (Towle and Godolphin, 2013).

Participation in Governance

Consumer participation in decisions about a provider organization's policy direction and management supports the development of psychosocial interventions that meet the needs of consumers (Grant, 2010; Taylor et al., 2009). Consumers' increasing assumption of decision-making roles in provider organizations and governmental bodies has resulted in innovations that have improved the quality of care (e.g., peer support services) (Allen et al., 2010). Consumer participation in managing services directly informs organizations about consumer needs and has been strongly associated with consumers' having information about service quality and how to access services (Omeni et al., 2014).

Consumer councils are common, and can be effective in involving clients in formal policy reviews and performance improvement projects (Taylor et al., 2009). Consumer council involvement provides staff with a better understanding of consumers' views and expectations, increases clients' involvement in service improvement, and can impact management decisions (Linhorst et al., 2005). Clients are more likely to participate when their program (e.g., group homes, hospitals) encourages their independence and involvement in decision making (Taylor et al., 2009).

Service Provision

By actively participating in discussions within treatment teams and with staff more generally, consumers bring a lived experience that can round out a more clinical view, improving the treatment decision-making process. Consumers take on a wide variety of service delivery roles as peer support workers, a general term applying to people with a lived experience of mental illness who are empathetic and provide direct emotional support for a consumer. Operating in these roles, peers can play an important part in quality management and transformation (Drake et al., 2010). In August 2007, the Centers for Medicare & Medicaid Services (CMS) issued a letter to state Medicaid directors designating peer support as a billable service and outlining the minimum requirements that should be addressed for this role (CMS, 2007).

Shared Decision Making and Decision Support Systems for Psychosocial Interventions

Shared decision making is a collaborative process through which patients and their providers make health care decisions together, taking into account patients' values and preferences and the best scientific evidence and patient data available (Drake et al., 2010). Key to this process are training individual providers in effective communication and supporting clients in openly expressing their service preferences.

Shared decision making has been found to be most effective when computer-based decision support systems are in place to assist providers in implementing clinical guidelines and clients in expressing treatment preferences and making informed decisions (Goscha and Rapp, 2014). These systems provide tailored assessments and evidence-based treatment recommendations for providers to consider based on patient information that is entered through an electronic health record (EHR) system (Deegan, 2010). On the consumer side, a software package elicits information from patients, at times guided by peer specialists, and prints out their goals and preferences in relation to their expressed needs and diagnosis. These systems also provide structural support to both consumers and clinicians in the care planning process—for example, through reminders for overdue services and screenings, recommendations for evidence-based psychosocial interventions, and recommendations for health behavior changes.

PROVIDERS

Behavioral health providers bring commitment and training to their work. Many, if not most, efforts to improve the quality of psychosocial interventions have focused on providers, reflecting their key role in helping clients achieve recovery and quality of life. Provider-focused efforts to improve quality of care include dissemination of treatment information, such as through manuals and guidelines; various forms of training, coaching, expert consultation, peer support, and supervision; fidelity checks; and provider profiling and feedback on performance. The Cochrane Effective Practice and Organisation of Care (EPOC) Group has conducted systematic reviews documenting the effectiveness of various provider-focused strategies for quality improvement, such as printed educational materials (12 randomized controlled trials [RCTs], 11 nonrandomized studies), educational meetings (81 RCTs), educational outreach (69 RCTs), local opinion leaders (18 RCTs), audit and feedback (118 RCTs), computerized remind- ers (28 RCTs), and tailored implementation (26 RCTs) (Cochrane, 2015; Grimshaw et al., 2012). Research on the implementation of evidence-based psychosocial interventions has focused overwhelmingly on strategies that entail monitoring fidelity (also referred to as adherence and compliance) and assessing provider attitudes toward or satisfaction with the interven- tions (Powell et al., 2014). Other clinician-level factors that can influence and improve quality include competence, motivation, and access to diag- nostic and decision-making tools. Importantly, as noted above with regard to consumers, providers actively working in clinical settings should be engaged in the quality improvement culture and the design and application of these levers.

Provider Education and Training

The delivery of quality mental health care requires a workforce ad- equately trained in the knowledge and skills needed for delivering evidence- based psychosocial interventions. For almost two decades, federal reports have emphasized the shortage of professionals who are trained to deliver evidence-based interventions (HHS, 1999; NIMH, 2006). Quality improve- ment of behavioral health care is thwarted by low awareness of evidence- based practices among providers (Brown et al., 2008), likely a result of the relatively low percentage of graduate training programs that require didactic or clinical supervision in evidence-based practices (Bledsoe et al., 2007; Weissman et al., 2006).

Several reviews have focused on the efficacy of different educational techniques used to train providers in evidence-based psychosocial treat- ments (e.g., Beidas and Kendall, 2010; Herschell et al., 2010; Rakovshik and McManus, 2010). While passive approaches (e.g., single-session workshops and distribution of treatment manuals) may increase providers' knowledge and even predispose them to adopt a treatment, such approaches do little to produce behavior change (Davis and Davis, 2009; Herschell et al., 2010). In contrast, effective education and training often involve multifaceted strate- gies, including a treatment manual, multiple days of intensive workshop training, expert consultation, live or taped review of client sessions, supervi- sor trainings, booster sessions, and the completion of one or more training cases (Herschell et al., 2010). Leaders in the field of provider training also have suggested that training should be dynamic and active and address a wide range of learning styles (Davis and Davis, 2009); utilize behavioral rehearsal (Beidas et al., 2014); and include ongoing supervision, consulta- tion, and feedback (Beidas and Kendall, 2010; Rakovshik and McManus, 2010). The effectiveness of training is dependent as well on such factors as workshop length, opportunity to practice skills, and trainer expertise. One issue limiting the utility of training as a lever for quality improvement is that training in psychosocial treatment often is proprietary, with training fees beyond the reach of many service organizations, particularly those serving safety net populations.

A number of studies have found that after learning a new intervention, clinicians do not use the intervention quickly or frequently enough to maintain skills in its delivery over time (Cross et al., 2014, 2015). Because there are no agreed-upon standards for postgraduate training methods and assessment of skill acquisition beyond a brief knowledge-based quiz, continuing education activities and postgraduate training and certification programs vary widely in content and method. Long-term effects of training also are dependent on the amount of posttraining support that is available. Checklists, introduced in the practice setting to prompt the delivery of treatment protocols, have been shown to be moderately successful in increasing providers' implementation of research-based practice recommendations (Albrecht et al., 2013).

Training programs can apply state-of-the-art adult learning practices at multiple levels (i.e., as part of degree-granting programs, postgraduate programs, and continuing education) to ensure that trainees are indeed adept at evidence-based psychosocial interventions. Considerable evidence supports models that include skill-building opportunities through observation of experts and practice with standardized cases (Chun and Takanishi, 2009; Cross et al., 2007; Matthieu et al., 2008; Wyman et al., 2008), access to expert consultation after training (Mancini et al., 2009), and ongoing peer support (Austin et al., 2006) to sustain skill sets. Two examples of postgraduate training in psychosocial interventions are the United Kingdom's Improving Access to Psychological Therapies (IAPT) program and the Veterans Health Administration's (VHA's) National Evidence-Based Psychotherapy Dissemination and Implementation Model.

In the early 2000s the United Kingdom's National Health Service (NHS) invested considerable funds in improving the mental health and well-being of U.K. citizens. As part of those efforts, the IAPT program, an independent, nongovernmental body consisting of experts in the various evidence-based psychotherapies, was created to prepare the workforce to provide evidence-based treatments for a variety of behavioral health problems. Although the program initially focused on training in cognitive-behavioral therapy, it has since added training in other interventions, including interpersonal psychotherapy; brief dynamic therapy; eye movement desensitization and reprocessing; mindfulness-based cognitive therapy; and family interventions for parenting, eating disorders, and psychosis (UCL, 2015). Two types of clinicians are trained: low-intensity therapists, who work with consumers suffering from mild to moderate depression and anxiety, and high-intensity therapists, who provide face-to-face psychotherapy for more severe illnesses or complex cases. The competencies and curricula for training in these models were developed jointly by NHS and professional organizations that historically have been involved in training clinicians in these practices.

Regardless of the intervention model, high-intensity therapists undergo 1 year of training, which consists of 2 days of coursework and 3 days of clinical service each week (NHS, 2015). Therapists in training are assigned cases involving the conditions for which the treatments are indicated, are supervised weekly, and provide videotapes of their therapeutic encounters that are rated by experts. Trainees must demonstrate competence in the interventions to be certified as high-intensity therapists. Low-intensity therapists undergo a similar training process, but need undergo only 8 months of training (Layard and Clark, 2014). Although not without its initial detractors, this training program has been highly successful. As of 2012, it had resulted in 3,400 new clinicians being capable of providing evidence-based interventions in the United Kingdom, which has translated into 1.134 million people being treated for mental health problems, two-thirds demonstrating "reliable" recovery, and 45 percent showing full remission (Department of Health, 2012). The IAPT creators note that intervention expert involvement and buy-in are critical to the success of the model.

In the United States, the VHA's National Evidence-Based Psychotherapy Dissemination and Implementation Model is an example of successful postgraduate training in evidence-based practices (see Box 6-1). The VHA also has achieved nationwide implementation of contingency management, an evidence-based treatment for substance abuse, through targeted trainings and ongoing implementation support (Petry et al., 2014). Like the United Kingdom, the VHA has been able to demonstrate enhanced quality of care provided to veterans, with clinicians showing improved clinical competencies and self-efficacy and greater appreciation for evidence-based treatments (Karlin and Cross, 2014b). These changes in practice also have led to improved clinical outcomes in patient populations (Karlin and Cross, 2014b). Since embarking on providing training and support in the delivery of evidence-based psychosocial interventions, the VHA has seen positive effects in suicidal ideation, posttraumatic stress disorder, and depression in veterans seeking care (Watts et al., 2014).

Although the efforts of the United Kingdom and the VHA to effect these changes in practice have resulted in positive outcomes, they were not without their problems. In the United Kingdom, an initial barrier to the IAPT program was having stakeholders agree to a national curriculum tied to practice guidelines. This problem was solved by actively involving professional organizations in detailing the competencies required and in creating tools with which to measure those competencies. Both the U.K. and VHA systems also suffer from long wait times to access treatment, largely because of the limited workforce equipped to provide evidence-based care.

BOX 6-1
An Example of In-field Provider Training in
Evidence-Based Practices: The Veterans Health
Administration's (VHA's) National Evidence-Based
Psychotherapy Dissemination and Implementation Model

In 2007, the VHA created and deployed a competency-based training program to train existing psychologists and social workers in evidence-based psychotherapies for mental health problems such as posttraumatic stress disorder and depression, and to ensure that therapists' competencies and skill levels would be maintained over time. The model consists of participation in an in-person workshop in which actual clinical skills are taught and practiced. The workshop is followed by 6 months of ongoing telephone consultation with experts in the evidence-based practices, as well as long-term local support to ensure sustained skills. By the end of fiscal year 2012, training had been provided to 6,400 VHA behavioral health clinicians (Karlin and Cross, 2014b). The program focused initially on cognitive-behavioral therapy but more recently has expanded to cover other evidence-based psychotherapies as well.

The process begins when regional mental health directors select providers to participate in a training organized by the VHA Central Office. In the skill-building workshop, trainers assess the providers' skills using standardized and validated competency checklists. The providers are then instructed to identify cases with which to practice the new intervention and receive weekly telephone-based support from an expert. Providers are given clinical tools, such as manuals, videos demonstrating the practices, and patient education tools. Once the ongoing support has been completed, the providers are offered virtual office hours, when experts are available to provide consultation on challenging cases. The long-term local support consists of peer consultation, available through groups called communities of practice, to foster organizational change and support the implementation of the new practices (Ranmuthugala et al., 2011a,b).

The program has shown positive training outcomes, such as increased clinical competencies, enhanced self-efficacy, and improved knowledge and attitudes. The program also has led to moderate to large improvements in patient outcomes (Karlin and Cross, 2014b).

However, studies have shown that wait times in the VHA are not substantially longer than those in other health services settings (Brandenburg et al., 2015).

CLINICAL SETTINGS AND PROVIDER ORGANIZATIONS

Behavioral health settings vary widely in organizational readiness and capacity for quality improvement (Aarons et al., 2012; Emmons et al.,

2012). Moreover, community settings for behavioral health care differ greatly from the controlled research settings where psychosocial treatments are developed and tested. Emerging evidence that effectiveness often declines markedly when interventions are moved from research to real-world settings (Schoenwald and Hoagwood, 2001) signals the need to address important ecological issues when designing and testing psychosocial treatments. Several advances in implementation science—such as hybrid research designs (Curran et al., 2012), principles of "designing for dissemination" (Brownson et al., 2012), and monitoring and ongoing adaptation to enhance quality (Chambers et al., 2013; Zayas et al., 2012)—offer promising ways to better fit psychosocial interventions to the real-world contexts in which behavioral health care is delivered.

A variety of organizational levers can enhance the quality of behavioral health care. Evidence-based care is facilitated by innovation champions within an organization and clear leadership support for quality analysis and improvement (Brown et al., 2008; Simpson and House, 2002). The implementation of evidence-based practices also is enhanced by management support for innovation, the availability of adequate financial resources, and a learning orientation within the organization (Klein and Knight, 2005). A particular leadership style—transformational leadership—is associated with a climate supportive of innovation and the adoption of evidence-based practices (Aarons and Sommerfeld, 2012). In a program for people with schizophrenia, for example, the implementation of evidence-based care was facilitated by a number of organization-level factors, including champions, provider incentives, intensive provider education, the addition of care managers, and information systems (Brown et al., 2008).

The Availability, Responsiveness, and Continuity (ARC) model is an example of a manualized multicomponent, team-based organizational strategy for quality care (Glisson and Schoenwald, 2005; Glisson et al., 2010). Designed to improve the organizational context in which services are provided, this model has been found effective in a wide range of mental health, health, and social service settings. Quality improvement collaboratives, including the Institute for Healthcare Improvement's Breakthrough Series Collaborative Model (Ebert et al., 2012; IHI, 2003), have proven helpful to organizations in implementing interventions for physical health conditions (Pearson et al., 2005). Further research is needed to determine the effectiveness of these collaboratives for the implementation of evidence-based care for behavioral health conditions. Specially designed technical support centers external to a given organization also can support quality improvement. External facilitation, used within the VHA to implement evidence-based psychotherapies, has been found to be effective, low-cost, feasible, and scalable (Kauth et al., 2005). Likewise, the Children's Bureau within the U.S. Department of Health and Human Services (HHS) funds five regional Implementation Centers within its Training and Technical Assistance Network to help states and tribes improve the quality of child welfare services, including, in some cases, the implementation of evidence-based programs (ACF, n.d.).

One clear challenge faced by organizations is the cost of quality improvement efforts, above and beyond those costs associated with the delivery of psychosocial treatment itself. The adoption of new treatments and quality improvement entail costs, such as those for training, consultation, and supervision; fidelity monitoring; and infrastructure changes associated with embedding standardized assessments into routine forms and databases. Most community-based settings operate under reimbursement mechanisms that rarely cover the costs of implementing new interventions (Raghavan, 2012). Raghavan and colleagues (2008) characterize these system antecedents or requisites for evidence-based care as the "policy ecology of implementation." The implementation of evidence-based practices requires, at the organizational level, policies that provide for the added marginal costs of treatments and support the learning of new treatments at the organizational and provider levels. Saldana and colleagues (2014) developed a tool for calculating implementation costs; the "COIN" tool provides a feasible template for mapping costs onto observable activities and examining important differences in implementation strategies for an evidence-based practice. One psychosocial intervention for behavioral problems among youth, for example, cost more to implement through a team-based approach than through individual provider implementation "as usual," although the team-based approach was more efficient in terms of time to implementation and expenditure of staff hours. Further research is needed to identify cost-effective implementation strategies, and at the payor or regulatory level, policies are needed to leverage contractual mechanisms, utilize provider and organizational profiling, and support outcome assessment (Raghavan et al., 2008).

Finally, although the assessment of barriers to implementation is important, the field would benefit from rigorous study of the implementation processes and specific strategies that lead to sustained adoption and delivery of evidence-based interventions.

PURCHASERS AND PLANS

Purchasers (including private employers and the government, in the case of insurance programs such as Medicare and Medicaid) and health plans have a number of levers available for encouraging quality improvement for psychosocial interventions. These levers include strategies targeting primarily consumers, such as enrollee benefit design, and those targeting primarily providers, such as utilization management, patient registries, provider payment methods, and provider profiling.

Enrollee Benefit Design

Benefit design is a key strategy used by purchasers and plans to influence the use of health care services, including psychosocial interventions. By affecting the quantity and types of services used, benefit design also can affect the quality of care (Choudhry et al., 2010).

A large literature dating back more than 40 years documents that health care utilization levels tend to be lower when individuals face high out-of-pocket costs. The RAND Health Insurance Experiment, an RCT of the impact of cost sharing on health care utilization and spending conducted in the 1970s and 1980s, found that use of health care services declined sharply as cost-sharing requirements increased (Manning et al., 1988); other nationally representative surveys have yielded similar findings (Horgan, 1985, 1986). Use of ambulatory mental health services was about twice as responsive to the out-of-pocket cost faced by an enrollee as the use of ambulatory general medical services (Manning et al., 1988). More recent studies, conducted after the introduction of managed care, likewise have documented lower use of behavioral health services associated with higher cost-sharing levels (Rice and Morrison, 1994). Benefit design also can distort treatment decision making if different types of services are covered at differing levels of generosity. For example, if a plan requires much lower cost sharing for pharmacological treatments than for psychosocial interventions, individuals may be more likely to seek the former treatments only.

Because of the relationship between cost sharing and service use, the recent movement toward high-deductible health plans, which require enrollees to pay a large deductible (anywhere from $1,000 to $5,000 or higher) before the plan covers any health care expenses, could cause some individuals to reduce or altogether forego their use of beneficial evidence-based psychosocial treatments for mental health and substance use disorders (Kullgren et al., 2010). The same is true for the shift on the part of some health plans from requiring enrollees to make flat copayments to requiring coinsurance (i.e., paying a percentage of the fee for a service) (Choudhry et al., 2010). In contrast, value-based insurance designs, which involve tailoring cost-sharing requirements to the cost-effectiveness of a given service in an effort to improve the value of care delivered (i.e., lower cost sharing for higher-value services), could result in more appropriate use of evidence-based psychosocial treatments (Eldridge and Korda, 2011).

Utilization Management

Plans use a variety of utilization management techniques to influence the use of health care services by members. A plan's goals for these techniques include controlling growth in health care spending and improving the quality of care—for example, by discouraging treatment overuse or misuse. Common utilization management techniques include prior authorization requirements, concurrent review, and fail-first policies (i.e., requiring an enrollee to "fail" on a lower-cost therapy before obtaining approval for coverage of a higher-cost therapy). These review processes can be burdensome for clinicians, and may encourage them to provide alternative treatments that are not subject to these techniques.

A large literature documents decreases in the use of health care services associated with utilization management techniques, with some studies suggesting that the quality of care could be adversely affected for some individuals (Newhouse et al., 1993). In the case of mental health–related prescription drugs, for example, the implementation of prior authorization requirements has been associated with reductions in the use of medications subject to prior authorization and lower medication expenditures, but also with reduced medication compliance and sometimes higher overall health care expenditures (e.g., Adams et al., 2009; Law et al., 2008; Lu et al., 2010; Motheral et al., 2004; Zhang et al., 2009). Similarly, the use of fail-first policies for prescription drugs (sometimes referred to as "step therapy") has been associated with lower prescription drug expenditures (e.g., Farley et al., 2008; Mark et al., 2010); however, one study of a fail-first policy for antidepressant medications found that adoption of this policy was associated with an increase in mental health–related inpatient admissions, outpatient visits, and emergency room visits for antidepressant users in affected plans (Mark et al., 2010). Thus, the use of these tools can have both intended and unintended outcomes, and these outcomes can be linked to quality of care. However, a carefully constructed utilization management strategy could serve to improve the quality of psychosocial interventions if it resulted in more appropriate use of these interventions among those most likely to benefit from them. On the other hand, as with benefit design, the differential application of utilization management across treatment modalities could affect treatment decision making (i.e., individuals might be less likely to use services subject to stricter utilization management).

Selective contracting and network management is another utilization management tool used by plans that can influence the provision of psychosocial interventions. Plans typically form exclusive provider networks, contracting with a subset of providers in the area. Under this approach, plans generally provide more generous coverage for services delivered by network providers than for those delivered by providers outside the network. As a result, plans often can negotiate lower fees in exchange for the patient volume that will likely result from being part of the plan's network. To ensure the availability of evidence-based psychosocial interventions, a plan's provider network must include adequate numbers of providers with skills in delivering these interventions who are accepting new patients. Importantly, plans will need tools with which to determine the competence of network providers in delivering evidence-based treatments. Network adequacy has been raised as a concern in the context of new insurance plans offered on the state-based health insurance exchanges under the Patient Protection and Affordable Care Act (Bixby, 1998).

As discussed in Chapter 1, the Mental Health Parity and Addiction Equity Act requires parity in coverage for behavioral health and general medical services. Parity is required in both quantitative treatment limitations (e.g., copays, coinsurance, inpatient day limits, outpatient visit limits) and nonquantitative treatment limitations, including the use of utilization management techniques by plans. Thus, plans are prohibited from using more restrictive utilization management for mental health and substance use services than for similar types of general medical services. However, the regulations would not govern differential use of utilization management techniques across different mental health/substance use treatment modalities (e.g., drugs versus psychosocial treatments).

Provider Payment

The methods used to pay health care providers for the services they deliver influence the types, quantity, and quality of care received by consumers. Historically, providers typically were paid on a fee-for-service (FFS) basis, with no explicit incentives for performance or quality of care. FFS payment creates incentives for the delivery of more services, as each service brings additional reimbursement, but does not encourage the coordination of care or a focus on quality improvement. Since their introduction more than 20 years ago, managed behavioral health care carve-outs—a dominant method of financing mental health/substance use care whereby specialty benefits for this care are separated from the rest of health care benefits and managed by a specialty managed care vendor—also have shaped the financing and delivery of behavioral health services. These arrangements allow the application of specialty management techniques for behavioral health care and help protect a pool of funds for behavioral health services (b⌐ a separate budget and contract are established just for these serv⌐ definition, however, carve-out contracts increase fragmentatio⌐ delivery and distort clinical decision making to some extent. ⌐ risk-based carve-out contracts have traditionally excluded p⌐ cations, giving carve-out organizations an incentive to e⌐

of medications over psychosocial interventions when the two types of interventions could otherwise be viewed as substitutable (Huskamp, 1999).

Over the past several years, two trends have been emerging: (1) a move away from FFS payment toward bundled payment arrangements, a form of risk-based payment under which providers face some level of financial risk for the health care expenditures of a given patient population; and (2) increasing use of pay-for-performance (P4P) approaches in provider contracts.

Bundled Payments

Instead of reimbursing each provider individually for every service delivered to a patient under an FFS model, bundled payment models involve fixed payments for bundles of related services. The bundle of services can be defined relatively narrowly (e.g., all physician and nonphysician services delivered during a particular inpatient stay) or more broadly, with the broadest bundle including all services provided to an individual over the course of a year (i.e., a global budget). The current Medicare accountable care organization (ACO) demonstration programs fall somewhere in the middle of this continuum, including almost all services in the bundle but placing the large provider organizations that serve as ACOs at only limited—not full—financial risk for total health care spending.

Bundled payment arrangements create incentives for efficiency in the delivery of all services included in the bundle and for greater coordination of care, in addition to providing incentives to substitute services not included in the bundle (and thus reimbursed outside of the bundled payment) where possible. These arrangements also raise concerns about stinting and poor quality of care to the extent that maintaining or improving quality can be costly. In the case of psychosocial interventions, there is concern that provider organizations operating under a global full risk payment contract, with strong incentives for efficiency in service delivery, could reduce the delivery of effective psychosocial interventions for which measurement of quality is problematic or there is no incentive for the provision of quality in payment systems, as is the case for many psychosocial interventions (Mechanic, 2012).

Pay-for-Performance (P4P)

Both public and private purchasers and plans also have embraced P4P approaches to encouraging quality improvement. Under P4P, clinicians or provider organizations receive bonuses if they meet or exceed certain quality thresholds that are specified in provider contracts. While the literature P4P strategies suggests that they often result in improved quality as measured by the metrics used, the improvements often are relatively small in magnitude and may be somewhat narrowly focused on the clinical areas that are targeted through the measures (Colla et al., 2012; Mullen et al., 2010; Werner et al., 2013; Wilensky, 2011).

Risk-based payment models currently in use for Medicare and some commercial payers include a P4P component, with a set of performance metrics and associated financial incentives. The P4P components are included in the risk-based contracts in an effort to ensure that quality of care is maintained or improved in the face of greater provider financial risk for expenditures. Given such financial risk, provider organizations may be more likely to discourage the use of treatments with no associated quality metrics or less focused on ensuring the quality of those treatments relative to treatments for which financial incentives are included in the contract. This concern underscores the importance of incorporating validated quality metrics for psychosocial treatments in P4P systems. For any metrics based on outcome measures, it will be important for the P4P methodology to account for differences in patient case mix to counteract incentives for selection behavior on the part of clinicians and provider organizations.

Provider Profiling and Public Reporting

The collection of data and issuance of periodic reports to providers on their performance relative to that of other providers in their practice setting, provider group, or overall plan or payer has been carried out in the medical arena for many years. Provider profiling is based on the premise that giving providers feedback that compares their performance with that of others will motivate them to improve in areas in which they may be underperforming. This is one strategy that could be incorporated into a quality improvement system adopted by providers, plans, and purchasers in an effort to improve the quality of psychosocial interventions.

Evidence on the effectiveness of profiling in the medical arena has been mixed. A review by the Cochrane Collaborative found evidence of improvement in clinical standards (Jamtvedt et al., 2006), although a later study found mixed evidence that provider profiling served as a catalyst for quality improvement activities (Fung et al., 2008).

An extension of provider profiling is the public reporting of information from provider profiles. Public reporting systems, such as Medicare's Nursing Home Compare and New York State's reporting system for cardiovascular disease providers, can include information at the organization level (e.g., hospital, group practice) or at the individual clinician level. In theory, public reporting can improve quality of care in two primary ways. First, by providing consumers and family members with information on the quality of care delivered by different clinicians or provider organizations, public reporting can facilitate consumer selection of high-quality providers. Second, public reporting of quality metrics can encourage individual clinicians and provider organizations to engage in efforts to improve the quality of care, both to protect their reputation and to attract new patients.

A literature review on public reporting of quality measures conducted by the Agency for Healthcare Research and Quality (AHRQ, 2012), however, found little or no effect of public reporting on provider selection by consumers and family members. Consumers often said they were unaware of the publicly reported data when making provider selection decisions, or that they found the reports confusing or lacking in key information needed for making a decision (AHRQ, 2012). On the other hand, the review found evidence of a positive effect of public reporting systems on the behavior of clinicians and provider organizations, including improvements in quality measures over time among profiled providers, increased focus on quality improvement activities, evidence that some surgeons with the worst outcomes left surgical practice, and hospitals offering new services in response to public reporting (AHRQ, 2012). The review also found that the impacts of public reporting appeared to be greater in more competitive versus less competitive health care markets (AHRQ, 2012).

As for P4P systems, provider profiling and public reporting systems must account for differences in patient case mix to counteract incentives for selection behavior on the part of clinicians and provider organizations.

REGULATORS OF TRAINING AND EDUCATION

In the United States, professional organizations (e.g., the American Psychiatric Association, the American Psychological Association, Council on Social Work Education) and associated accreditation and certification organizations (e.g., the Accreditation Council for Graduate Medical Education, the American Board of Psychiatry and Neurology) and state licensing and accreditation agencies determine the competencies that professional schools are required to teach their students, and evaluate the success of the schools based on a set of predetermined standards. For example, the American Psychological Association accredits graduate programs and clinical internships based on each program's ability to document successes in graduation, the percentage who become licensed, and whether the program teaches basic core competencies (APA, n.d.). In its new accreditation standards, still in the public comment stage, the American Psychological Association calls on doctoral training programs to focus on "empirically supported intervention procedures." Likewise, the 2008 accreditation standards of the Council on Social Work Education require that social work trainees "employ evidence-based interventions." The Accreditation Council for Graduate Medical Education and the American Board of Psychiatry and Neurology require, as a condition of accreditation, that residents be trained in cognitive-behavioral therapy and that they be able to summarize the evidence base for that therapy; the same requirements now apply as well to psychodynamic psychotherapy and supportive psychotherapies (ACGME and ABPN, 2013). Nonetheless, these efforts by professional and accrediting bodies are nascent; even when these bodies require that students, residents, and fellows be trained in evidence-based practices, programs are given little guidance as to which practices are indeed evidence based, what models of training are most effective, or how the acquisition of core competencies should be assessed. As a result, accredited training programs vary considerably in the degree to which they offer training in evidence-based practices. If professional and accrediting organizations are to exert greater leadership in ensuring effective training in evidence-based practices, they will need to reach consensus on the competencies needed to implement those practices and on the best means of determining that a training program is successfully preparing its students in their delivery. This approach has been used successfully in training models developed by IAPT and the VHA. In the United States, professional organizations and intervention authors and experts could work together to create a competence framework, as well as ensure that the training methods are effective and that those trained can demonstrate competence.

At the postgraduate and continuing education level, providers are required in many states to accrue continuing education credits to maintain licensure. Providers are known to value training in evidence-based practices that accords with their clients' needs, that offers continuing education opportunities, and that is advanced beyond the "beginning level" (Powell et al., 2013). Continuing education as required by state licensing or professional certification organizations thus can be used as a lever for quality improvement. As with professional schools, state professional organizations may need to determine whether a continuing education activity meets quality standards for adult learning and establish clear guidance on what competencies may need to be renewed.

MULTILEVEL QUALITY IMPROVEMENT AND IMPLEMENTATION

A growing body of research demonstrates the effectiveness of quality improvement efforts focused on each of the stakeholders discussed in this chapter. Yet growing evidence suggests that multifaceted implementation strategies targeting multiple levels of service provision—consumers, providers, organizations, payers, and regulators—are most effective. For example, effective implementation of acceptance and commitment therapy was shown to require multilevel, coordinated efforts on the part of state mental health authorities, senior program administrators, and program staff (Proctor et al., 2009). High-fidelity implementation of the therapy was facilitated by dedicated billing mechanisms, technical assistance centers, and program monitoring (Mancini et al., 2009). Yet while some studies testing comprehensive or blended strategies have shown positive effects (Forsner et al., 2010; Glisson et al., 2010), the same is true for more narrowly focused strategies (Herschell et al., 2010; Lochman et al., 2009). With more than 60 different implementation strategies being reported in the literature (Powell et al., 2012), encompassing planning, training, financing, restructuring, management, and policy approaches, research is needed to identify the most effective, efficient, and parsimonious approaches. The National Institutes of Health (NIH) has designated as a priority effort to "identify, develop, and refine effective and efficient methods, structures, and strategies to disseminate and implement" innovations in health care (NIH, 2009).

Improving the quality of psychosocial interventions is a particular need (Goldner et al., 2011; Herschell et al., 2010). For instance, a scoping review of the published literature focused on implementation research in mental health identified 22 RCTs, only 2 of which tested psychosocial interventions in mental health settings (Goldner et al., 2011). This finding stands in contrast to the broader field of health care, in which the number of RCTs testing implementation strategies dwarfs the number in mental health and social service settings. This differential led Landsverk and colleagues (2011) to conclude that the field of mental health has lagged behind other disciplines in building an evidence base for implementation.

CONCLUSION AND RECOMMENDATIONS

This chapter and the report as a whole have described the need to consider quality not as a binary, static characteristic but as existing within a complex context and as part of a cycle of actions leading to the implementation of quality improvement by the multiple stakeholders involved in the delivery of care for mental health and substance use disorders. These stakeholders—from consumers who receive psychosocial interventions; to the providers who render the interventions; to their clinics and the organizations in which the clinics are embedded; to payers, regulators, and policy makers—each have levers, incentives, and other means by which they can move the system toward higher quality. These contextual factors and levers interact with one another in complex ways, and the means by which their effects occur are not yet fully understood. Much of the evidence surrounding the use of these levers to improve quality is weak but promising, and needs to be augmented with further research.

The committee drew the following conclusion about improving the quality of psychosocial interventions:

Multiple stakeholders should apply levers, incentives, and other means to create learning health systems that continually progress toward higher quality (as recommended in previous IOM Quality Chasm reports).

Recommendation 6-1. *Adopt a system for quality improvement.* Purchasers, plans, and providers should adopt systems for measuring, monitoring, and improving quality for psychosocial interventions. These systems should be aligned across multiple levels. They should include structure, process, and outcome measures and a combination of financial and nonfinancial incentives to ensure accountability and encourage continuous quality improvement for providers and the organizations in which they practice. Quality improvement systems also should include measures of clinician core competencies in the delivery of evidence-based psychosocial interventions. Public reporting systems, provider profiling, pay-for-performance, and other accountability approaches that include outcome measures should account for differences in patient case mix (e.g., using risk adjustment methods) to counteract incentives for selection behavior on the part of clinicians and provider organizations, especially those operating under risk-based payment.

Recommendation 6-2. *Support quality improvement at multiple levels using multiple levers.* Purchasers, health care insurers, providers, consumers, and professional organizations should pursue strategies designed to support the implementation and continuous quality improvement of evidence-based psychosocial interventions at the provider, clinical organization, and health system levels.

- The infrastructure to support high-quality treatment includes ongoing provider training, consumer and family education, supervision, consultation, and leadership to enhance organizational culture and foster a climate for continuously learning health care systems. Other core aspects of infrastructure for the implementation and quality improvement of evidence-based psychosocial interventions include the use of registries, electronic health records, and computer-based decision support systems for providers and consumers, as well as technology-supported technical assistance and training.
- This infrastructure could be fostered by a nonprofit organization, supported and funded through a public–private partnership (e.g., the Institute for Healthcare Improvement), that would provide technical assistance to support provider organizations and clinicians in quality improvement efforts.

Recommendation 6-3. *Conduct research to design and evaluate strategies that can influence the quality of psychosocial interventions.* Research is needed to inform the design and evaluation of policies, organizational levers, and implementation/dissemination strategies that can improve the quality of psychosocial interventions and health outcomes. Potential supporters of this research include federal, state, and private entities.

- Policies should be assessed at the patient, provider, clinical organization/system, payer, purchaser, and population levels.
- Examples might include research to develop and assess the impact of benefit design changes and utilization management tools, new models of payment and delivery, systems for public reporting of quality information, and new approaches for training in psychosocial interventions.

REFERENCES

Aarons, G. A., and D. H. Sommerfeld. 2012. Leadership, innovation climate, and attitudes toward evidence-based practice during a statewide implementation. *Journal of the American Academy of Child and Adolescent Psychiatry* 51(4):423-431.

Aarons, G., J. Horowitz, L. Dlugosz, and M. Ehrhart. 2012. The role of organizational processes in dissemination and implementation research. In *Dissemination and implementation research in health: Translating science to practice,* by R. Brownson, G. A. Colditz, Enola K. Proctor. New York: Oxford University Press. Pp. 128-153.

ACF (Administration for Children and Families). n.d. *Training and technical assistance.* http://www.acf.hhs.gov/programs/cb/assistance (accessed January 1, 2015).

ACGME (Accreditation Council for Graduate Medical Education) and ABPN (American Board of Psychiatry and Neurology). 2013. *The psychiatry milestone project.* http://acgme.org/acgmeweb/Portals/0/PDFs/Milestones/PsychiatryMilestones.pdf (accessed June 17, 2015).

Adams, A. S., F. Zhang, R. F. LeCates, A. J. Graves, D. Ross-Degnan, D. Gilden, T. J. McLaughlin, C. Lu, C. M. Trinacty, and S. B. Soumerai. 2009. Prior authorization for antidepressants in Medicaid: Effects among disabled dual enrollees. *Archives of Internal Medicine* 169(8):750-756.

AHRQ (Agency for Healthcare Research and Quality). 2012. *Closing the quality gap series: Public reporting as a quality improvement strategy.* http://www.effectivehealthcare.ahrq.gov/search-for-guides-reviews-and-reports/?pageaction=displayproduct&productID=1198 (accessed June 17, 2015).

Albrecht, L., M. Archibald, D. Arseneau, and S. D. Scott. 2013. Development of a checklist to assess the quality of reporting of knowledge translation interventions using the Workgroup for Intervention Development and Evaluation Research (WIDER) recommendations. *Implementation Science* 8(52).

Allen, J., A. Q. Radke, and J. Parks. 2010. *Consumer involvement with state mental health authorities.* Alexandria, VA: National Association of Consumer/Survivor Mental Health Administrators.

APA (American Psychological Association). n.d. *Understanding APA accreditation.* http://www.apa.org/ed/accreditation/about (accessed June 17, 2015).

Austin, Z., A. Marini, N. MacLeod Glover, and D. Tabak. 2006. Peer-mentoring workshop for continuous professional development. *American Journal of Pharmaceutical Education* 70(5):117.

Barbato, A., B. D'Avanzo, V. D'Anza, E. Montorfano, M. Savio, and C. G. Corbascio. 2014. Involvement of users and relatives in mental health service evaluation. *The Journal of Nervous and Mental Disease* 202(6):479-486.

Beidas, R. S., and P. C. Kendall. 2010. Training therapists in evidence-based practice: A critical review of studies from a systems contextual perspective. *Clinical Psychology: Science and Practice* 17:1-30.

Beidas, R. S., W. Cross, and S. Dorsey. 2014. Show me, don't tell me: Behavioral rehearsal as a training and analogue fidelity tool. *Cognitive and Behavioral Practice* 21(1):1-11.

Bixby, T. D. 1998. Network adequacy: The regulation of HMO's network of health care providers. *Missouri Law Review* 63:397.

Bledsoe, S. E., M. M. Weissman, E. J. Mullen, K. Ponniah, M. Gameroff, H. Verdeli, L. Mufson, H. Fitterling, and P. Wickramaratne. 2007. Empirically supported psychotherapy in social work training programs: Does the definition of evidence matter? *Research on Social Work Practice* 17:449-455.

Brandenburg, L., P. Gabow, G. Steele, J. Toussaint, and B. Tyson. 2015. *Innovation and best practices in health care scheduling.* Discussion paper. Washington, DC: Institute of Medicine. http://www.iom.edu/schedulingbestpractices (accessed June 15, 2015).

Brown, A. H., A. N. Cohen, M. J. Chinman, C. Kessler, and A. S. Young. 2008. EQUIP: Implementing chronic care principles and applying formative evaluation methods to improve care for schizophrenia: QUERI Series. *Implementation Science* 3:9.

Brownson, R. C., J. A. Jacobs, R. G. Tabak, C. M. Hoehner, and K. A. Stamatakis. 2012. Designing for dissemination among public health researchers: Findings from a national survey in the United States. *American Journal of Public Health* 103(9):1693-1699.

Chambers, D. A., R. E. Glasgoe, and K. C. Stange. 2013. The dynamic sustainability framework: Addressing the paradox of sustainment amid ongoing change. *Implementation Science* 8:117.

Choudhry, N. K., M. B. Rosenthal, and A. Milstein. 2010. Assessing the evidence for value-based insurance design. *Health Affairs* 29(11):1988-1994.

Chun, M. B., and D. M. Takanishi, Jr. 2009. The need for a standardized evaluation method to assess efficacy of cultural competence initiatives in medical education and residency programs. *Hawaii Medical Journal* 68(1):2-6.

Clark, C. C., E. A. Scott, K. M. Boydell, and P. Goering. 1999. Effects of client interviewers on client-reported satisfaction with mental health services. *Psychiatric Services* 50(7):961-963.

CMS (Centers for Medicare & Medicaid Services). 2007. *Letter to state Medicaid directors.* SMDL #07-011. August 15, 2007. http://downloads.cms.gov/cmsgov/archived-downloads/SMDL/downloads/SMD081507A.pdf (accessed June 16, 2015).

Cochrane. 2015. *Cochrane effective practice and organisation of care group: Our reviews.* http://epoc.cochrane.org/our-reviews (accessed June 18, 2015).

Colla, C. H., D. E. Wennberg, E. Meara, J. S. Skinner, D. Gottlieb, V. A. Lewis, C. M. Snyder, and E. S. Fisher. 2012. Spending differences associated with the Medicare Physician Group Practice Demonstration. *Journal of the American Medical Association* 308(10):1015-1023.

Cross, W., M. M. Matthieu, J. Cerel, and K. L. Knox. 2007. Proximate outcomes of gatekeeper training for suicide prevention in the workplace. *Suicide and Life-Threatening Behavior* 37(6):659-670.

Cross, W. F., A. R. Pisani, K. Schmeelk-Cone, Y. Xia, X. Tu, M. McMahon, J. L. Munfakh, and M. Gould. 2014. Measuring trainer fidelity in the transfer of suicide prevention training. *Crisis* 35(3):202-212.

Cross, W., J. West, P. A. Wyman, K. Schmeelk-Cone, Y. Xia, X. Tu, M. Teisl, C. H. Brown, and M. Forgatch. 2015. Observational measures of implementer fidelity for a school-based preventive intervention: Development, reliability, and validity. *Prevention Science: The Official Journal of the Society for Prevention Research* 16(1):122-132.

Curran, G. M., M. Bauer, B. Mittman, J. M. Pyne, and C. Stetler. 2012. Effectiveness-implementation hybrid designs: Combining elements of clinical effectiveness and implementation research to enhance public health impact. *Medical Care* 50(3):217-226.

Davis, D. A., and N. Davis. 2009. Educational interventions. In *Knowledge translation in health care: Moving from evidence to practice*, edited by S. Straus, J. Tetroe, and I. D. Graham. Oxford, England: Wiley-Blackwell. Pp. 113-123.

Deegan, P. E. 2010. A web application to support recovery and shared decision making in psychiatric medication clinics. *Psychiatric Rehabilitation Journal* 34(1):23-28.

Delman, J. 2007. Consumer-driven and conducted survey research in action. In *Towards best practices for surveying persons with disabilities*, Vol. 1, edited by T. Kroll, D. Keer, P. Placek, J. Cyril, and G. Hendershot. Hauppauge, NY: Nova Publishers. Pp. 71-87.

Delman, J., and A. Lincoln. 2009. Service users as paid research workers: Principles for active involvement and good practice guidance. In *Handbook of service user involvement in mental health research*, edited by J. Wallcraft, B. Schrank, and M. Amering, New York: John Wiley & Sons, Ltd. Pp. 139-151.

Department of Health (U.K.). 2012. *IAPT three-year report: The first million patients.* http://www.iapt.nhs.uk/silo/files/iapt-3-year-report.pdf (accessed June 17, 2015).

Drake, R. E., P. E. Deegan, and C. Rapp. 2010. The promise of shared decision making in mental health. *Psychiatric Rehabilitation Journal* 34(1):7-13.

Ebert, L., L. Amaya-Jackson, J. M. Markiewicz, C. Kisiel, and J. A. Fairbank. 2012. Use of the breakthrough series collaborative to support broad and sustained use of evidence-based trauma treatment for children in community practice settings. *Administration and Policy in Mental Health* 39(3):187-199.

Eldridge, G. N., and H. Korda. 2011. Value-based purchasing: The evidence. *American Journal of Managed Care* 17(8):e310-e313.

Emmons, K. M., B. Weiner, M. E. Fernandez, and S. P. Tu. 2012. Systems antecedents for dissemination and implementation: A review and analysis of measures. *Health Education and Behavior* 39(1):87-105.

Farley, J. F., R. R. Cline, J. C. Schommer, R. S. Hadsall, and J. A. Nyman. 2008. Retrospective assessment of Medicaid step-therapy prior authorization policy for atypical antipsychotic medications. *Clinical Therapeutics* 30(8):1524-1539.

Forsner, T., A. A. Wistedt, M. Brommels, I. Janszky, A. P. de Leon, and Y. Forsell. 2010. Supported local implementation of clinical guidelines in psychiatry: A two year follow-up. *Implementation Science* 5:1-11.

Fung, C. H., Y. W. Lim, S. Mattke, C. Damberg, and P. G. Shekelle. 2008. Systematic review: The evidence that publishing patient care performance data improves quality of care. *Annals of Internal Medicine* 148(2):111-123.

Glisson, C., and S. K. Schoenwald. 2005. The ARC organizational and community intervention strategy for implementing evidence-based children's mental health treatments. *Mental Health Services Research* 7(4):243-259.

Glisson, C., S. K. Schoenwald, A. Hemmelgarn, P. Green, D. Dukes, K. S. Armstrong, and J. E. Chapman. 2010. Randomized trial of MST and ARC in a two-level evidence-based treatment implementation strategy. *Journal of Consulting and Clinical Psychology* 78(4):537-550.

Goldner, E. M., V. Jeffries, D. Bilsker, E. Jenkins, M. Menear, and L. Petermann. 2011. Knowledge translation in mental health: A scoping review. *Healthcare Policy* 7:83-98.

Goscha, R., and C. Rapp. 2014. Exploring the experiences of client involvement in medication decisions using a shared decision making model: Results of a qualitative study. *Community Mental Health Journal* 1-8.

Grant, J. G. 2010. Embracing an emerging structure in community mental health services hope, respect, and affection. *Qualitative Social Work* 9(1):53-72.

Grimshaw, J. M., M. P. Eccles, J. N. Lavis, S. J. Hill, and J. E. Squires. 2012. Knowledge translation of research findings. *Implementation Science* 7:1-17.

Herschell, A. D., D. J. Kolko, B. L. Baumann, and A. C. Davis. 2010. The role of therapist training in the implementation of psychosocial treatments: A review and critique with recommendations. *Clinical Psychology Review* 30:448-466.

HHS (U.S. Department of Health and Human Services). 1999. *Mental health: A report of the Surgeon General.* Rockville, MD: HHS, Substance Abuse and Mental Health Services Administration, Center for Mental Health Services, National Institutes of Health, National Institute of Mental Health.

Hibbard, J. H. 2013. What the evidence shows about patient activation: Better health outcomes and care experiences; fewer data on costs. *Health Affairs* 32(2):207.

Horgan, C. M. 1985. Specialty and general ambulatory mental health services: A comparison of utilization and expenditures. *Archives of General Psychiatry* 42:565-572.

_____. 1986. The demand for ambulatory mental health services from specialty providers. *Health Services Research* 21(2):291-319.

Huskamp, H. A. 1999. Episodes of mental health and substance abuse treatment under a managed behavioral health care carve-out. *Inquiry* 36(2):147-161.

IHI (Institute for Healthcare Improvement). 2003. *The breakthrough series: IHI's collaborative model for achieving breakthrough improvement.* http://www.ihi.org/resources/Pages/IHIWhitePapers/TheBreakthroughSeriesIHIsCollaborativeModelforAchievingBreakthroughImprovement.aspx (accessed June 17, 2015).

IOM (Institute of Medicine). 2006. *Improving the quality of care for mental and substance use conditions.* Washington, DC: The National Academies Press.

Jamtvedt, G., J. M. Young, D. T. Kristoffersen, M. A. O'Brien, and A. D. Oxman. 2006. Audit and feedback: Effects on professional practice and health care outcomes. *Cochrane Database of Systematic Reviews* (2):CD000259.

Karlin, B. E., and G. Cross. 2014a. Enhancing access, fidelity, and outcomes in the national dissemination of evidence-based psychotherapies. *American Psychologist* 69(7):709-711.

_____. 2014b. From the laboratory to the therapy room: National dissemination and implementation of evidence-based psychotherapies in the U.S. Department of Veterans Affairs health care system. *American Psychologist* 69(1):19-33.

Kauth, M. R., G. Sullivan, and K. L. Henderson. 2005. Supporting clinicians in the development of best practice innovations in education. *Psychiatric Services* 56(7):786-788.

Klein, K. J., and A. P. Knight. 2005. Innovation implementation: Overcoming the challenge. *Current Directions in Psychological Science* 14(5):243-246.

Kullgren, J. T., A. A. Galbraith, V. L. Hinrichsen, I. Miroshnik, R. B. Penfold, M. B. Rosenthal, B. E. Landon, and T. A. Lieu. 2010. Health care use and decision making among lower-income families in high-deductible health plans. *Archives of Internal Medicine* 170(21):1918-1925.

Landsverk, J., C. H. Brown, J. Rolls Reutz, L. A. Palinkas, and S. M. Horwitz. 2011. Design elements in implementation research: A structured review of child welfare and child mental health studies. *Administration and Policy in Mental Health* 38:54-63.

Law, M. R., D. Ross-Degnan, and S. B. Soumerai. 2008. Effect of prior authorization of second-generation antipsychotic agents on pharmacy utilization and reimbursements. *Psychiatric Services* 59(5):540-546.

Layard, R., and D. M. Clark. 2014. *Thrive: How better mental health care transforms lives and saves money*. Princeton, NJ: Princeton University Press.

Linhorst, D. M., and A. Eckert. 2002. Involving people with severe mental illness in evaluation and performance improvement. *Evaluation & The Health Professions* 25(3):284-301.

Linhorst, D. M., A. Eckert, and G. Hamilton. 2005. Promoting participation in organizational decision making by clients with severe mental illness. *Social Work* 50(1):21-30.

Lochman, J. E., N. P. Powell, C. L. Boxmeyer, L. Qu, K. C. Wells, and M. Windle. 2009. Implementation of a school-based prevention program: Effects of counselor and school characteristics. *Professional Psychology: Research and Practice* 40(5):476.

Lu, C. Y., S. B. Soumerai, D. Ross-Degnan, F. Zhang, and A. S. Adams. 2010. Unintended impacts of a Medicaid prior authorization policy on access to medications for bipolar illness. *Medical Care* 48(1):4-9.

Mancini, A. D., L. L. Moser, R. Whitley, G. J. McHugo, G. R. Bond, M. T. Finnerty, and B. J. Burns. 2009. Assertive community treatment: Facilitators and barriers to implementation in routine mental health settings. *Psychiatric Services* 60(2):189-195.

Manning, W. G., J. P. Newhouse, N. Duan, E. B. Keeler, B. Benjamin, A. Liebowitz, and M. S. Marquis. 1988. *Health insurance and the demand for medical care: Evidence from a randomized experiment*. Report R-3476-HHS. Santa Monica, CA: RAND Corporation.

Mark, T. L., T. M. Gibson, K. McGuigan, and B. C. Chu. 2010. The effects of antidepressant step therapy protocols on pharmaceutical and medical utilization and expenditures. *American Journal of Psychiatry* 167(10):1202-1209.

Matthieu, M. M., W. Cross, A. R. Batres, C. M. Flora, and K. L. Knox. 2008. Evaluation of gatekeeper training for suicide prevention in veterans. *Archives of Suicide Research: Official Journal of the International Academy for Suicide Research* 12(2):148-154.

Mechanic, D. 2012. Seizing opportunities under the Affordable Care Act for transforming the mental and behavioral health system. *Health Affairs* 31(2):376-382.

Motheral, B. R., R. Henderson, and E. R. Cox. 2004. Plan-sponsor savings and member experience with point-of-service prescription step therapy. *American Journal of Managed Care* 10:457-464.

Mullen, K. J., R. G. Frank, and M. B. Rosenthal. 2010. Can you get what you pay for? Pay-for-performance and the quality of healthcare providers. *The RAND Journal of Economics* 41(1):64-91.

Newhouse, J. P., and the Insurance Experiment Group. 1993. *Free for All? Lessons from the RAND Health Insurance Experiment*. Cambridge, MA: Harvard University Press.

NHS (U.K. National Health Service). 2015. *High intensity cognitive behavioural therapy workers*. http://www.iapt.nhs.uk/workforce/high-intensity (accessed June 16, 2015).

NIH (National Institutes of Health). 2009. *Dissemination and implementation research in health (R03)*. Funding Opportunity Announcement PAR-10-039. http://grants.nih.gov/grants/guide/pa-files/PAR-10-039.html (accessed June 17, 2015).

NIMH (National Institute of Mental Health). 2006. *The road ahead: Research partnerships to transform services*. http://www.nimh.nih.gov/about/advisory-boards-and-groups/namhc/reports/road-ahead_33869.pdf (accessed June 16, 2015).

Omeni, E., M. Barnes, D. MacDonald, M. Crawford, and D. Rose. 2014. Service user involvement: Impact and participation: A survey of service user and staff perspectives. *BMC Health Services Research* 14(1):491.

Pearson, M. L., S. Wu, J. Schaefer, A. E. Bonomi, S. M. Shortell, P. J. Mendel, J. A. Marsteller, T. A. Louis, M. Rosen, and E. B. Keeler. 2005. Assessing the implementation of the chronic care model in quality improvement collaboratives. *Health Services Research* 40(4):978-996.

Petry, N. M., D. DePhilippis, C. J. Rahs, M. Drapkin, and J. R. McKay. 2014. Nationwide dissemination of contingency management: The Veterans Administration Initiative. *The American Journal on Addictions* 23:205-210.

Powell, B. J., J. C. McMillen, E. K. Proctor, C. R. Carpenter, R. T. Griffey, A. C. Bunger, J. E. Glass, and J. L. York. 2012. A compilation of strategies for implementing clinical innovations in health and mental health. *Medical Care Research and Review* 69(2):123-157.

Powell, B. J., J. C. McMillen, K. M. Hawley, and E. K. Proctor. 2013. Mental health clinicians' motivation to invest in training: Results from a practice-based research network survey. *Psychiatric Services* 64(8):816-818.

Powell, B. J., E. K. Proctor, and J. E. Glass. 2014. A systematic review of strategies for implementing empirically supported mental health interventions. *Research on Social Work Practice* 24(2):192-212.

Proctor, E. K., J. Landsverk, G. Aarons, D. Chambers, C. Glisson, and B. Mittman. 2009. Implementation research in mental health services: An emerging science with conceptual, methodological, and training challenges. *Administration and Policy in Mental Health and Mental Health Services Research* 36:24-34.

Raghavan, R. 2012. The role of economic evaluation in dissemination and implementation research. In *Dissemination and implementation research in health*, Ch. 5, edited by R. C. Brownson, G. A. Colditz, and E. K. Proctor. New York: Oxford University Press. Pp. 94-113.

Raghavan, R., C. L. Bright, and A. L. Shadoin. 2008. Toward a policy ecology of implementation of evidence-based practices in public mental health settings. *Implementation Science* 3:26.

Rakovshik, S. G., and F. McManus. 2010. Establishing evidence-based training in cognitive behavioral therapy: A review of current empirical findings and theoretical guidance. *Clinical Psychology Review* 30:496-516.

Ranmuthugala, G., F. C. Cunningham, J. J. Plumb, J. Long, A. Georgiou, J. I. Westbrook, and J. Braithwaite. 2011a. A realist evaluation of the role of communities of practice in changing healthcare practice. *Implementation Science* 6:49.

Ranmuthugala, G., J. J. Plumb, F. C. Cunningham, A. Georgiou, J. I. Westbrook, and J. Braithwaite. 2011b. How and why are communities of practice established in the healthcare sector? A systematic review of the literature. *BMC Health Services Research* 11:273.

Rice, T., and K. R. Morrison. 1994. Patient cost sharing for medical services: A review of the literature and implications for health care reform. *Medical Care Research and Review* 51(3):235-287.

Saldana, L., P. Chamberlain, W. D. Bradford, M. Campbell, and J. Landsverk. 2014. The Cost of Implementing New Strategies (COINS): A method for mapping implementation resources using the stages of implementation completion. *Children and Youth Services Review* 39:177-182.

Schoenwald, S. K. and K. Hoagwood. 2001. Effectiveness, transportability, and dissemination of interventions: What matters when? *Psychiatric Services* 52(9):1190-1197.

Simpson, E. L., and A. O. House. 2002. Involving service users in delivery and evaluation of mental health services: Systematic review. *British Medical Journal* 325:1265-1271.

Taylor, T. L., H. Killaspy, C. Wright, P. Turton, S. White, T. W. Kallert, M. Schuster, J. A. Cervilla, P. Brangier, J. Raboch, L. Kalisová, G. Onchev, H. Dimitrov, R. Mezzina, K. Wolf, D. Wiersma, E. Visser, A. Kiejna, P. Piotrowski, D. Ploumpidis, F. Gonidakis, J. Caldas-de-Almeida, G. Cardoso, and M. B. King. 2009. A systematic review of the international published literature relating to quality of institutional care for people with longer term mental health problems. *BMC Psychiatry* 9(1):55.

Towle, A., and W. Godolphin. 2013. Patients as educators: Interprofessional learning for patient-centred care. *Medical Teacher* 35(3):219-225.

Towle, A., L. Bainbridge, W. Godolphin, A. Katz, C. Kline, B. Lown, I. Madularu, P. Solomon, and J. Thistlethwaite. 2010. Active patient involvement in the education of health professionals. *Medical Education* 44(1):64-74.

Turnbull, P. and F. Weeley. 2013. Service user involvement: Inspiring student nurses to make a difference to patient care. *Nurse Education in Practice* 13(5):454-458.

UCL (University College London). 2015. *UCL competence frameworks for the delivery of effective psychological interventions.* https://www.ucl.ac.uk/pals/research/cehp/research-groups/core/competence-frameworks (accessed June 16, 2015).

Watts, B. V., B. Shiner, L. Zubkoff, E. Carpenter-Song, J. M. Ronconi, and C. M. Coldwell. 2014. Implementation of evidence-based psychotherapies for posttraumatic stress disorder in VA specialty clinics. *Psychiatric Services* 65(5):648-653.

Weissman, M. M., H. Verdeli, M. J. Gameroff, S. E. Bledsoe, K. Betts, L. Mufson, H. Fitterling, and P. Wickramaratne. 2006. National survey of psychotherapy training in psychiatry, psychology, and social work. *Archives of General Psychiatry* 63(8):925-934.

Werner, R. M., R. T. Konetzka, and D. Polsky. 2013. The effect of pay-for-performance in nursing homes: Evidence from state Medicaid programs. *Health Services Research* 48(4):1393-1414.

Wilensky, G. R. 2011. ACO regs, round 1. *Healthcare Financial Management: Journal of the Healthcare Financial Management* 65(5):30, 32.

Wyman, P. A., C. H. Brown, J. Inman, W. Cross, K. Schmeelk-Cone, J. Guo, and J. B. Pena. 2008. Randomized trial of a gatekeeper program for suicide prevention: 1-year impact on secondary school staff. *Journal of Consulting and Clinical Psychology* 76(1):104-115.

Zayas, L. H., J. L. Bellamy, and E. K. Proctor. 2012. Considering the multiple service contexts in cultural adaptations of evidence-based practices. In *Dissemination and implementation research in health,* edited by R. C. Brownson, G. A. Colditz, and E. K. Proctor. New York: Oxford University Press. Pp. 483-497.

Zhang, Y., A. S. Adams, D. Ross-Degnan, F. Zhang, and S. B. Soumerai. 2009. Effects of prior authorization on medication discontinuation among Medicaid beneficiaries with bipolar disorder. *Psychiatric Services (Washington, D.C.)* 60(4):520-527.

Appendix A

Data Sources and Methods

The Institute of Medicine (IOM) Committee on Developing Evidence-Based Standards for Psychosocial Interventions for Mental Disorders was tasked with developing a framework for the establishment of efficacy standards for psychosocial interventions used to treat individuals with mental disorders (inclusive of addictive disorders). The committee also explored strategies that different stakeholders might use to help establish these standards for psychosocial treatments. To respond comprehensively to its charge, the committee examined data from a variety of sources, including a review of the literature, open-session meetings and conference calls, public testimony and input, and other publicly available resources. The study was contracted over an 18-month period.

COMMITTEE EXPERTISE

The IOM formed a committee of 16 experts to conduct a study to respond to the study charge. The committee comprised members with expertise in health care policy, health care quality and performance, health systems research and operation, implementation science, intervention development and evaluation, primary care, professional education, clinical psychology and psychiatry, recovery-oriented care, and peer support services. Appendix B provides biographical information for each committee member.

LITERATURE REVIEW

Several strategies were used to identify literature relevant to the committee's charge. A search of bibliographic databases, including PubMed, SCOPUS, and Web of Science, was conducted to obtain articles from peer-reviewed journals. Staff reviewed recent literature on psychosocial care to identify articles relevant to the committee's charge and created an End-Note database. In addition, committee members, meeting participants, and members of the public submitted articles and reports on these topics. The committee's database included more than 300 relevant articles and reports.

PUBLIC MEETINGS

The committee deliberated from March 2014 through December 2014 to conduct this expert assessment. During this period, the committee held five 2-day meetings, and committee members also participated in multiple conference calls. Two public meetings were held in conjunction with the committee's May and July 2014 meetings, which allowed committee members to obtain additional information on specific aspects of the study charge (see Boxes A-1 and A-2).

The first public meeting focused on approaches to quality measurement both in and outside the mental health care field. The second public meeting focused on approaches to quality improvement both in and outside the mental health care field, and included speakers with expertise in the fields of treatment fidelity, implementation, and health technology.

Each open-session meeting included a public comment period in which the committee invited input from any interested party. All open-session meetings were held in Washington, DC. A conference call number and online public comment tool were provided to allow opportunity for input from those unable to travel to the meetings. A link to the public comment tool was made available on the National Academies' website from January 2014 to March 2015, and all online comments were catalogued in the study's public access file. Any information provided to the committee from outside sources or through the online comment tool is available by request through the National Academies' Public Access Records Office. The agendas for the two open-session committee meetings are presented below.

BOX A-1
Agenda for Public Workshop on Quality Measurement

Keck Center, Room 101
The National Academies
500 Fifth Street, NW
Washington, DC

May 19, 2014

1:00 p.m. **Welcome and Introductions**
Mary Jane England, M.D., *Chair*

1:10 p.m. **Panel Discussion: Broad Issues in Quality Measurement**
Sarah Hudson Scholle, Dr.P.H., M.P.H., *Panel Moderator*

Helen Burstin, M.D., M.P.H.
Senior Vice President for Performance Measures
National Quality Forum

Shari M. Ling, M.D.
Deputy Chief Medical Officer
Center for Clinical Standards and Quality
Centers for Medicare & Medicaid Services

Eric C. Schneider, M.S., M.D.
Senior Scientist
Distinguished Chair in Health Care Quality
RAND Corporation

2:10 p.m. **Panel Discussion: Measuring Quality in Behavioral Health Services**
Kermit Crawford, Ph.D., *Panel Moderator*

Gregory J. McHugo, Ph.D.
Professor of Community and Family Medicine and of Psychiatry
Associate Director, Dartmouth Psychiatric Research Center
Dartmouth University

Kimberly Hepner, Ph.D.
Senior Behavioral Scientist
RAND Corporation

continued

BOX A-1 Continued

Jodie Trafton, Ph.D.
Director, VA Program Evaluation and Resource Center, Office of
Mental Health Operations, U.S. Department of Veterans Affairs
Health Science Specialist, Center for Innovation to
Implementation, VA Palo Alto

Jim Chase, M.A.
President
MN Community Measurement

3:10 p.m. Break

3:30 p.m. Panel Discussion: Measuring Quality in Other Fields
Harold Pincus, M.D, *Panel Moderator*

Matthew M. Hutter, M.D.
Assistant Professor in Surgery, Harvard Medical School
Associate Visiting Surgeon, Massachusetts General Hospital

Frank G. Opelka, M.D., FACS
President and Chief Executive, Louisiana State University
Healthcare Network
Associate Medical Director, American College of Surgeons
Division of Advocacy and Health Policy
Chair, American Medical Association–convened Physician
Consortium for Performance Improvement

Kurt C. Stange, M.D., Ph.D.
Promoting Health Across Boundaries
Editor, Annals of Family Medicine
Professor of Family Medicine and Community Health,
Epidemiology and Biostatistics, Oncology and Sociology
Case Western Reserve University

Kevin Larsen, M.D.
Medical Director of Meaningful Use
Office of the National Coordinator for Health Information
Technology
U.S. Department of Health and Human Services

4:30 p.m. Discussion

5:00 p.m. Adjourn

BOX A-2
Agenda for Public Workshop on Quality Improvement

Keck Center, Room 101
The National Academies
500 Fifth Street, NW
Washington, DC

July 23, 2014

1:00 p.m. **Welcome and Introductions**
Mary Jane England, M.D., *Chair*

1:10 p.m. **SAMHSA Criteria for Evaluating Evidence-Based Psychosocial**
Treatments

Lisa C. Patton, Ph.D.
Branch Chief, Quality, Evaluation, and Performance
Center for Behavioral Health Statistics and Quality
Substance Abuse and Mental Health Services Administration
(SAMHSA)

1:30 p.m. **Panel Discussion: Implementation**
Enola Proctor, Ph.D., *Panel Moderator*

Tracey L. Smith, Ph.D.
Mental Health Services, VA Central Office, Washington, DC

Virna Little, Psy.D., LCSW-R, SAP
Institute for Family Health

Abe Wandersman, Ph.D.
University of South Carolina

Gregory Aarons, Ph.D.
University of California, San Diego

2:40 p.m. **Panel Discussion: Treatment Fidelity**
Rhonda Robinson-Beale, M.D., *Panel Moderator*

Amy Dorin, LCSW
Federation Employment and Guidance Service (FEGS)

Sonja Schoenwald, Ph.D.
Medical University of South Carolina

continued

BOX A-2 Continued

David Clark, D.Phil., CBE, FBA, FMedSci, HonFBPs
Improving Access to Psychological Therapies (IAPT)

3:50 p.m. Break

4:00 p.m. Panel Discussion: Health IT
Sarah Hudson Scholle, Dr.P.H., M.P.H., *Panel Moderator*

David Mohr, Ph.D.
Northwestern University

Robert Gibbons, Ph.D.
University of Chicago

Armen Arevian, M.D., Ph.D.
University of California, Los Angeles

Grant Grissom, Ph.D.
Polaris Health Directions

4:30 p.m. Discussion

5:00 p.m. Adjourn

July 24, 2014

9:00 a.m. Health Reform and the Implications for Psychosocial Interventions

Richard Frank, Ph.D.
Assistant Secretary for Planning and Evaluation (ASPE)
U.S. Department of Health and Human Services

10:00 a.m. Adjourn

Appendix B

Committee Member Biographies

Mary Jane England, M.D. (*Chair*), is professor of health policy and management at the Boston University School of Public Health. Recently, she successfully completed a term as interim chair of community health sciences at the Boston University School of Public Health. In 1964, Dr. England received her medical degree from Boston University and launched an international career as a child psychiatrist. As an authority on employer and employee benefits, she has brought multiple informed perspectives to bear on health care reform. She was the first commissioner of the Massachusetts Department of Social Services (1979-1983), associate dean and director of the Littauer Master in Public Administration Program at the John F. Kennedy School of Government at Harvard University (1983-1987), president of the American Medical Women's Association (1986-1987), president of the American Psychiatric Association (1995-1996), and a corporate vice president of Prudential (1987-1990) and chief executive officer (CEO) of the Washington Business Group on Health (1990-2001). A nationally known expert on health care and mental health parity, Dr. England chaired the Institute of Medicine (IOM) committee that produced the 2006 Quality Chasm report on care for mental health and substance use disorders. In 2008, she chaired an IOM committee on parental depression and its effect on children and other family members. In 2011, she chaired an IOM committee on the public health dimensions of the epilepsies. Having recently completed a term on the Commission on Effective Leadership (2006-2009) of the American Council on Education and currently participating in the Advancing Care Together project in Colorado (2009-present), Dr. England continues to serve on Mrs. Rosalynn Carter's Task Force on Mental Health at the Carter Center. As president of Regis College (2001-2011), she oversaw a number of transformations, including taking the undergraduate women's college into coeducation; building its graduate programs, notably in nursing, health administration, and other health professions; and developing curricula to serve the needs of diverse populations of 21st-century students through interdisciplinary pathways.

Susan M. Adams, Ph.D., RN, PMHNP, FAANP, is professor of nursing and faculty scholar for community engaged behavioral health at Vanderbilt University School of Nursing and a licensed psychiatric mental health nurse practitioner (PMHNP). A respected advanced practice psychiatric nurse and educator, Dr. Adams served as program director for Vanderbilt's PMHNP program for almost two decades, developing a modified distance option program and overseeing its sustained growth and national recognition. Her research with community partners such as The Next Door, an agency that serves women with substance abuse problems reentering the community from incarceration, informs agency development and evaluation of new service lines, including trauma-informed care, on-site psychiatric medication management, supported employment, housing options, and family reintegration. Since 1997, Dr. Adams has served on the board of the Mental Health Cooperative, a multisite network that provides a continuum of services for individuals and families with serious mental illness. During her career, she has been a leader in clinical practice, education, and innovative models of care, with recent efforts in integration of primary care and behavioral health care. She has served on national panels and initiatives for the American Nurses Association (ANA), American Nurses Credentialing Center (ANCC), National Organization of Nurse Practitioner Faculties (NONPF), American Psychiatric Nurses Association (APNA), International Society of Psychiatric-Mental Health Nurses (ISPN) developing PMHNP competencies, the initial PMHNP certification exam, nurse practitioner faculty and program standards, and the PMH workforce. A frequent speaker at national conferences, Dr. Adams shares her expertise on co-occurring mental health and substance use disorders, screening and brief intervention for alcohol/drug abuse, fetal alcohol spectrum disorders (FASDs), PMHNP education for full scope of practice, and PMHNP certification review courses. Recent publications address treatment outcomes for co-occurring disorders, predictors of treatment retention, and training for nurses regarding FASD screening and prevention, as well as book chapters in widely used nursing texts on psychotherapeutic approaches for addictions and related disorders and on evidence-based practice. As current president of the APNA (2014-2015), Dr. Adams is focusing on collaboration initiatives that facilitate integrated models of care, interprofessional education, and research.

Patricia A. Areán, Ph.D., is a professor and director of targeted treatment development in the Department of Psychiatry and Behavioral Sciences at the University of Washington and is a licensed clinical psychologist. Dr. Areán is an international expert on the effectiveness of behavioral interventions for mood disorders. She leads a research and training group that is known for developing, studying, increasing access to, and implementing user-friendly, high-quality behavioral interventions for mood as it presents in chronic illness, aging, and low-income and ethnic minority populations and in a variety of service settings—mental health, primary care, senior services, and mobile platforms. Her team combines the latest information from cognitive neuroscience, socioeconomics, and implementation science in its designs. Since 1994, Dr. Areán has published 115 peer-reviewed articles on these topics and has been funded by the Substance Abuse and Mental Health Services Administration (SAMHSA), the National Institute of Mental Health (NIMH), the National Institute on Aging (NIA), the National Institute of Diabetes and Digestive and Kidney Diseases (NIDDK), and the Hartford Foundation. She is currently funded by NIMH to study the effect of "brain games" and of mobile health apps on mood. Her work has won national recognition, resulting in an early career award from the American Psychological Association, a mid-career award from the National Institutes of Health (NIH) for her work on disseminating evidence-based practices, and the Award for Achievements in Diversity in Mental Health from the American Association of Geriatric Psychiatry. Dr. Areán currently leads an interdisciplinary research and implementation team consisting of researchers from diverse backgrounds, including social work, nursing, psychiatry, family and general medicine, medical sociology, and clinical psychology. She also provides training in evidence-based treatments to community mental health and health professionals, and is developing deployable and cost-effective training models based on contemporary adult learning methods.

John S. Brekke, Ph.D., is Frances G. Larson professor of social work research at the University of Southern California (USC) School of Social Work. He completed his Ph.D. in social welfare at the University of Wisconsin–Madison under the supervision of Dr. Mary Ann Test. He began his research career with the Program of Assertive Community Treatment project in Madison. He began as faculty at USC in 1984, and has taught research and clinical courses in the master of social work program and Ph.D. courses on treatment outcome research and research grant writing. Prior to assuming an academic appointment, Dr. Brekke held a number of clinical positions working with persons diagnosed with severe and persistent mental illness in inpatient and outpatient settings. Since 1989, he has been the principal investigator on numerous grants funded by NIMH—one from SAMHSA, one funded by the Patient-Centered Outcomes Research Institute

(PCORI), and two sponsored by the UniHealth Foundation. In 2010 he was awarded a 3-year Investigator Award in Health Policy Research from the Robert Wood Johnson Foundation. His work, focused on the improvement of community-based services for individuals diagnosed with severe mental illness, has integrated biological aspects of mental disorder into psychosocial rehabilitation for individuals with schizophrenia. Dr. Brekke has tested biosocial models for understanding rehabilitative outcomes in schizophrenia and has studied how to facilitate the implementation of evidence-based practices in community-based services for individuals with schizophrenia. He also serves as principal investigator on a project that has developed and manualized and is testing the effectiveness of a community-based peer health navigator intervention linking mental health and health services for the seriously mentally ill in behavioral health care settings.

Michelle G. Craske, Ph.D., is professor of psychology, psychiatry, and biobehavioral sciences and director of the Anxiety Disorders Research Center at the University of California, Los Angeles (UCLA). She has published extensively in the area of fear and anxiety disorders. In addition to many research articles, she has written academic books on the topics of the etiology and treatment of anxiety disorders, gender differences in anxiety, translation from the basic science of fear learning to the understanding and treating of phobias, and principles and practice of cognitive-behavioral therapy, as well as several self-help books and therapist guides. In addition, she has been the recipient of NIMH funding since 1993 for research projects pertaining to risk factors for anxiety disorders and depression among children and adolescents, the cognitive and physiological aspects of anxiety and panic attacks, neural mediators of behavioral treatments for anxiety disorders, fear extinction mechanisms of exposure therapy, implementation of treatments for anxiety and related disorders, and constructs of positive and negative valence underlying anxiety and depression. She was associate editor for the *Journal of Abnormal Psychology*, and is presently associate editor for *Behaviour Research and Therapy* and *Psychological Bulletin*, as well as a scientific board member for the Anxiety and Depression Association of America. Dr. Craske was a member of the *Diagnostic and Statistical Manual of Mental Disorders*, Fourth Edition (DSM-IV) Anxiety Disorders Work Group and the DSM-5 Anxiety, Obsessive Compulsive Spectrum, Posttraumatic, and Dissociative Disorders Work Group (chair, Anxiety Disorders Subworkgroup). She is also a member of the American Psychological Association's Clinical Treatment Guidelines Advisory Steering Committee. Dr. Craske has given invited keynote addresses at many international conferences and frequently is invited to present training workshops on the most recent advances in cognitive-behavioral treatment for anxiety disorders. She is currently a professor in the Department of Psychology and Department of Psychiatry and Biobehavioral Sciences, UCLA, and director of the UCLA Anxiety Disorders Research Center. Dr. Craske received her B.A. Hons. from the University of Tasmania and her Ph.D. from the University of British Columbia.

Kermit Anthony Crawford, Ph.D., is a licensed psychologist and a designated forensic psychologist. He is director of the Center for Multicultural Mental Health (CMMH) and associate professor in the Division of Psychiatry at the Boston University School of Medicine. Dr. Crawford has expertise in mental health, psychology training, substance abuse, and workforce development and extensive experience in disaster behavioral health response and mental health training. He is principal investigator for several state and federal research and training grants. He has several publications in refereed journals and was recently lead author of a book chapter on the culturally competent practice of disaster behavioral health services. In addition to his earned doctorate from Boston College, Dr. Crawford is the recipient of an honorary doctoral degree of humane letters from the Massachusetts School of Professional Psychology. He has facilitated and provided disaster behavioral health response training across the nation on behalf of SAMHSA and the Federal Emergency Management Agency (FEMA). He provided consultation and training to disaster behavioral health responders in Mississippi and provided consultation and evaluation services in Louisiana in the aftermath of Hurricanes Rita and Katrina. He directed a team of behavioral health clinicians providing services to the evacuees from New Orleans, for which he was interviewed by the American Psychological Association's monthly publication *The Monitor on Psychology*. In his career, Dr. Crawford is committed to spanning cultures and to providing quality equitable mental health and behavioral health services to diverse underserved populations. He is also a psychologist with the New England Patriots.

Frank Verloin deGruy III, M.D., MSFM, is Woodward-Chisholm professor and chair of the Department of Family Medicine at the University of Colorado. He has held academic appointments at the Departments of Family Medicine at Case Western Reserve University, Duke University, and the University of South Alabama College of Medicine. A member of the IOM, he is past president of the Collaborative Family Healthcare Association and past president of the North American Primary Care Research Network. He currently serves on several national boards, including those of the National Network of Depression Centers (NNDC), the Council of Academic Family Medicine Organizations, the National Integration Academy Council (chair), and the Family Physicians' Inquiries Network (chair). His local activities involve board service for the 2040 Partners for Health organization and the

Colorado Institute of Family Medicine, as well as active service on a number of committees for the University of Colorado and the Anschutz Medical Campus. Dr. deGruy has authored more than 150 papers, chapters, books, and editorials, and has reviewed more than 1,000 grant applications for NIMH, the Agency for Healthcare Research and Quality (AHRQ), and the Robert Wood Johnson Foundation. He is currently on the editorial boards of *Families, Systems and Health*, the *Annals of Family Medicine*, and the *Primary Care Companion* to the *Journal of Clinical Psychiatry*.

Jonathan Delman, Ph.D., J.D., M.P.H., is an assistant research professor of psychiatry at the University of Massachusetts Medical School's Systems and Psychosocial Advances Research Center (SPARC). At SPARC, he is director of the Program for Recovery Research and associate director for participatory action research at the Transitions (to adulthood) Research and Training Center. He is also a senior researcher at the Technical Assistance Collaborative, a national housing and human services consulting firm. Dr. Delman is considered a national expert in recovery-oriented care and measurement, peer support services, community-based participatory action research (CBPR), and activating consumer participation in treatment decisions and policy development. He has regularly advised SAMHSA, NIMH, state agencies, peer organizations, and managed care companies on these matters. Additionally, he serves on several national health-related measurement and quality improvement committees. Dr. Delman is a mental health consumer researcher and a 2008 recipient of a Robert Wood Johnson Foundation Community Health Leader award, 1 of 10 awarded nationally, for "individuals who overcome daunting obstacles to improve health and health care in their communities." He was recognized for generating the development of a young adult voice in mental health research and policy, resulting in an altered service system landscape that now recognizes the unique service and support needs of young adults with behavioral health conditions.

Constance M. Horgan, Sc.D., is a professor at the Heller School for Social Policy and Management at Brandeis University and is the founding director of its Institute for Behavioral Health. From 2007 to 2013, she served as associate dean for research. Dr. Horgan's expertise is in health policy analysis and services research. Specifically, her research is focused on how alcohol, drug, and mental health services are financed, organized, and delivered in the public and private sectors and what approaches can be used to improve the quality and effectiveness of the delivery system. Dr. Horgan has led studies for a range of federal agencies (AHRQ, NIMH, the National Institute on Alcohol Abuse and Alcoholism [NIAAA], the National Institute on Drug Abuse [NIDA], SAMHSA); state government; and foundations, including the Robert Wood Johnson Foundation. She directed the Brandeis/ Harvard Center to Improve the Quality of Drug Abuse Treatment, funded by NIDA, which is focused on how performance measurement and management and payment techniques can be harnessed more effectively and efficiently to deliver higher-quality substance abuse treatment. For the past 15 years, Dr. Horgan has led a series of NIH-funded nationally representative surveys of the provision of behavioral health care in private health plans, including the use of incentives, performance measures, and other approaches to quality improvement, and how behavioral health parity legislation is affecting those services. She is a co-investigator on studies funded by NIDA, the Robert Wood Johnson Foundation, and the Centers for Medicare & Medicaid Services (CMS) on the design, implementation, and evaluation of provider and patient incentive payments to improve care delivery. For more than 20 years, Dr. Horgan has directed the NIAAA training program to support doctoral students in health services research, teaching core courses in the substance use and treatment areas and directing the weekly doctoral seminar. Currently, she is a member of the National Committee for Quality Assurance's (NCQA's) Behavioral Health Care Measurement Advisory Panel and also serves on the National Quality Forum's (NQF's) Behavioral Health Standing Committee. Dr. Horgan received her doctorate in health policy and management from Johns Hopkins University and her master's degree in demography from Georgetown University.

Haiden A. Huskamp, Ph.D., is a professor of health care policy in the Department of Health Care Policy at Harvard Medical School. She is a health economist with extensive experience studying utilization, spending, and quality of mental health and substance use disorder treatment through quantitative analysis of large administrative databases and qualitative analysis involving structured key informant interviews. Through grants from NIH and several private foundations, Dr. Huskamp is currently examining the effects of new payment and delivery models on mental health and substance use disorder treatment; the impact of federal mental health parity legislation; the design, implementation, and impacts of recent efforts to extend health insurance coverage to individuals involved in the criminal justice system; and factors influencing physician adoption of new antipsychotic medications. She co-directs a Harvard Medical School health policy course that is required of all first-year medical students. Dr. Huskamp previously served on the IOM committees on pediatric palliative care and on accelerating rare disease research and the development of orphan products.

Harold Alan Pincus, M.D., is professor and vice chair of the Department of Psychiatry at Columbia University's College of Physicians and Surgeons, director of quality and outcomes research at New York-Presbyterian

Hospital, and co-director of Columbia's Irving Institute for Clinical and Translational Research. Dr. Pincus is also a senior scientist at the RAND Corporation. Previously, he was director of the RAND-University of Pittsburgh Health Institute and executive vice chairman of the Department of Psychiatry at the University of Pittsburgh. He is national director of the Health and Aging Policy Fellows Program (funded by Atlantic Philanthropies and the John A. Hartford Foundation), and directed the Robert Wood Johnson Foundation's National Program on Depression in Primary Care and the John A. Hartford Foundation's national program on Building Interdisciplinary Geriatric Research Centers. Dr. Pincus was also deputy medical director of the American Psychiatric Association and founding director of its Office of Research. He served as special assistant to the director of NIMH and, as a Robert Wood Johnson Foundation clinical scholar, on the White House and congressional staffs. Among other recent projects, he led the national evaluation of mental health services for veterans, the redesign of primary care/behavioral health relationships in New Orleans, an NIH-funded national study of research mentoring, and evaluations of major federal and state programs to integrate health and mental health/substance abuse care. Dr. Pincus chairs the World Health Organization/*International Classification of Diseases* (ICD)-11 Technical Advisory Group on Quality and Patient Safety, the NQF Behavioral Health Standing Committee, and the Medicaid Task Force for the Measurement Applications Partnership under the Affordable Care Act.

Enola K. Proctor, Ph.D., is Shanti K. Khinduka distinguished professor at the Brown School of Social Work at Washington University in St. Louis. She is founding director of the Center for Mental Health Services Research at the George Warren Brown School of Social Work at Washington University in St. Louis. Since 1993, the Center has collaborated with its national network of research partners to build a base of evidence designed to address the challenges of delivering mental health services to vulnerable populations. Dr. Proctor's work to improve depression care to older adults has been supported by grants from NIMH, NIA, and private foundations. She is a national leader in the scientific study of the movement of evidence-based practices from clinical knowledge to practical applications. Dr. Proctor directs the Center for Dissemination and Implementation at Washington University's Institute for Public Health, along with research cores for dissemination and implementation research, including that for Washington University's Institute for Clinical and Translational Science. Her teaching focuses on service system and implementation science methods for social work, health, and mental health care settings. A generous and committed teacher to doctoral and master's students, she has led Washington University's NIMH-funded doctoral and postdoctoral training program in mental health services research for 20 years. She also leads the NIMH-funded Implementation Research Institute, a national training program for implementation science for mental health services. Her peer-reviewed publications address the quality of mental health services and the implementation of evidence-based interventions. Among her books are *Dissemination and Implementation Research in Health: Translating Science to Practice*, published in 2012 by Oxford University Press, and *Developing Practice Guidelines for Social Work Interventions: Issues, Methods, and Research Agenda*, published in 2003 by Columbia University Press. Dr. Proctor was a member of NIMH's National Advisory Council from 2007 to 2011 and served on two National Advisory Committee workgroups—on research workforce development and intervention research. She served as editor-in-chief of the research journal of the National Association of Social Workers, *Social Work Research*. Her awards include the Knee Wittman Award for Lifetime Achievement in Health and Mental Health Practice, National Association of Social Workers Foundation; the Distinguished Achievement Award from the Society for Social Work and Research; the President's Award for Excellence in Social Work Research, National Association of Social Workers; and Mental Health Professional of the Year, Alliance for the Mentally Ill of Metropolitan St. Louis. Along with university mentoring awards, she received Washington University's top honor, the Arthur Holly Compton Faculty Achievement Award. She also was elected as a founding member of the American Academy of Social Work and Social Welfare.

Rhonda Robinson-Beale, M.D., is senior vice president and chief medical officer at Blue Cross of Idaho. She was most recently chief medical officer for OptumHealth Behavioral Solutions, a leading provider of solutions for mental health and substance use disorders in California. Dr. Robinson-Beale developed quality initiatives and clinical systems for OptumHealth Behavioral Solutions. She has more than 20 years of experience in behavioral health and quality management and is an active member of the behavioral health community. She has been involved with NCQA as a surveyor; a member of the Review Oversite Committee, which makes accreditation decisions; and a member of advisory panels that developed the managed behavioral health care organization and disease management standards. She has also been a member of the board of directors for the IOM's Neuroscience and Behavioral Health and Health Care Services Boards and has served on several IOM committees. Dr. Robinson-Beale participated on NQF's board of directors as co-chair for the Evidence-Based Practices to Treat Substance Use Disorders Steering Committee. Before joining OptumHealth Behavioral Solutions, she was chief medical officer for PacifiCare Behavioral Health. She also served as senior vice president and chief medical officer for CIGNA Behavioral Health, national medical director for Blue Cross Blue

Shield, executive medical director of medical and care management clinical programs for Blue Cross Blue Shield of Michigan, and senior medical director for behavioral medicine for Health Alliance Plan. Dr. Robinson-Beale received her medical degree from Wayne State University and her psychiatric training at Detroit Psychiatric Institute. She is certified in psychiatry by the American Board of Psychiatry and Neurology.

Sarah Hudson Scholle, Dr.P.H., M.P.H., is a health services researcher and has responsibility for overseeing the development and implementation of NCQA's research agenda. Her research interests focus on assessing the quality of health care and understanding consumer perceptions and preferences in health care, particularly for women and families. Dr. Scholle leads efforts to develop new approaches to quality measurement and evaluation of health care, including comprehensive well care for children and women, care coordination for vulnerable populations, and patient experiences with the medical home. Her prior work supported the development of NCQA's recognition program for patient-centered medical homes and distinction programs for multicultural health care populations, as well as numerous quality measures. Prior to joining NCQA, Dr. Scholle served as associate professor at the University of Pittsburgh School of Medicine. She has numerous publications in major health services and women's health journals. She chairs a Health Services Research Merit Review Board for the Veterans Health Administration Health Services Research and Development Program. She also reviews manuscripts for a variety of journals (including *Health Services Research* and *Women's Health Issues*). She has served on expert panels for the IOM and NQF. Dr. Scholle received her bachelor's degree in history and master's degree in public health from Yale University and her doctorate in public health from the Johns Hopkins University School of Hygiene and Public Health.

John T. Walkup, M.D., is professor of psychiatry, DeWitt Wallace senior scholar, vice chair of psychiatry, and director of the Division of Child and Adolescent Psychiatry, Weill Cornell Medical College and New York-Presbyterian Hospital. Prior to joining the faculty at Weill Cornell, Dr. Walkup spent 20 years at Johns Hopkins School of Medicine serving as professor of psychiatry and behavioral sciences and deputy director in the Division of Child and Adolescent Psychiatry. He held a joint appointment in the Center for American Indian Health at the Johns Hopkins Bloomberg School of Public Health, where he was director of behavioral research. Dr. Walkup has three main academic areas of interest: his work with Tourette's syndrome uniquely spans psychiatry, child psychiatry, and neurology; his expertise in interventions research focuses on the development and evaluation of psychopharmacological and psychosocial treatments for the major psychiatric disorders of childhood, including anxiety, depression, bipolar disorder, Tourette's syndrome, and suicidal behavior; and lastly, he has been involved in developing and evaluating interventions to reduce the large mental health disparities facing Native American youth, specifically with respect to drug use and suicide prevention. Dr. Walkup was awarded the Norbert and Charlotte Rieger Award for Academic Achievement in 2009 from the American Academy of Child and Adolescent Psychiatry and the Blanche F. Ittleson Award for Research in Child Psychiatry in 2011 from the American Psychiatric Association. His team at the Center for American Indian Health at Johns Hopkins won the Bronze Achievement Award from the Institute of Psychiatric Services of the American Psychiatric Association in 2012 for a pioneering suicide prevention project on the White Mountain Apache Reservation. Dr. Walkup serves on the scientific advisory boards of the Trichotillomania Learning Center, the Anxiety Disorders Association of America, and the American Foundation of Suicide Prevention. He is also deputy editor for psychopharmacology for the *Journal of the American Academy of Child and Adolescent Psychiatry*. His research has been published in major medical journals, including the *Journal of the American Medical Association* and the *New England Journal of Medicine*.

Myrna Weissman, Ph.D., is Diane Goldman Kemper family professor of epidemiology in psychiatry, College of Physicians and Surgeons and Mailman School of Public Health at Columbia University, and chief of the Division of Epidemiology at New York State Psychiatric Institute. She is a member of the Sackler Institute for Developmental Psychobiology at Columbia. Until 1987, she was a professor of psychiatry and epidemiology at Yale University School of Medicine and director of the Depression Research Unit. She has been a visiting senior scholar at the IOM. Dr. Weissman's research focuses on understanding the rates and risks of mood and anxiety disorders using methods of epidemiology, genetics, and neuroimaging and the application of these findings to develop and test empirically based treatments and preventive interventions. Her current interest is in bringing psychiatric epidemiology closer to translational studies in the neurosciences and genetics. She directs a three-generation study of families at high and low risk for depression who have been studied clinically for more than 25 years and who are participating in genetic and imaging studies. She directs a multicenter study to determine the impact of maternal remission from depression on offspring. She also is one of the principal investigators for a multicenter study to find biomarkers of response to the treatment of depression. Dr. Weissman was one of the developers of interpersonal psychotherapy, an evidence-based treatment for depression. She is a member of the IOM. In April 2009, she was selected by the American College of Epidemiology as 1 of 10 epidemiologists in the United States who has had a major impact on public policy and public health. The summary of her work on depression appears in a special issue of the *Annals of Epidemiology, Triumphs in Epidemiology*. Dr. Weissman received a Ph.D. in epidemiology from Yale University School of Medicine in 1974.